THE ALPHABET

of the

HUMAN HEART

ROBINSON

First published in Australia in 2009 by Pan Macmillan Australia, a division of Macmillan

First published in the UK in 2009 by Robinson

A CIP catalogue record for this book
is available from the British Library.

ISBN: 978-1-84901-449-6

Printed and bound in Italy by Rotolito Lombardo SpA

Robinson
An imprint of
Little, Brown Book Group
Carmelite House
50 Victoria Embankment
London EC4Y 0DZ

An Hachette UK Company
www.hachette.co.uk

www.littlebrown.co.uk

Important Note
This book is not intended as a substitute for medical advice or treatment. Any person with a condition requiring medical attention should consult a medical practitioner or suitable therapist.

FOR OUR CHILDREN

FOR WHEN THEY GROW UP

Matthew Johnstone and James Kerr have helped each other through the upside and the downside of life for over 30 years. This book is the result of their friendship.

Please visit us at
www.alphaheart.com

THE ALPHABET
of the
HUMAN HEART

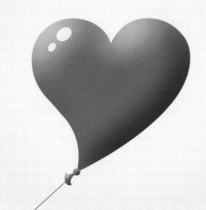

The A to Zen of Life

By Matthew Johnstone and James Kerr

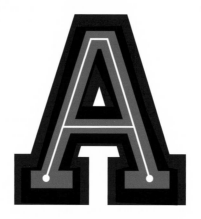

is for **adventure**

Adventure is the opposite of television.

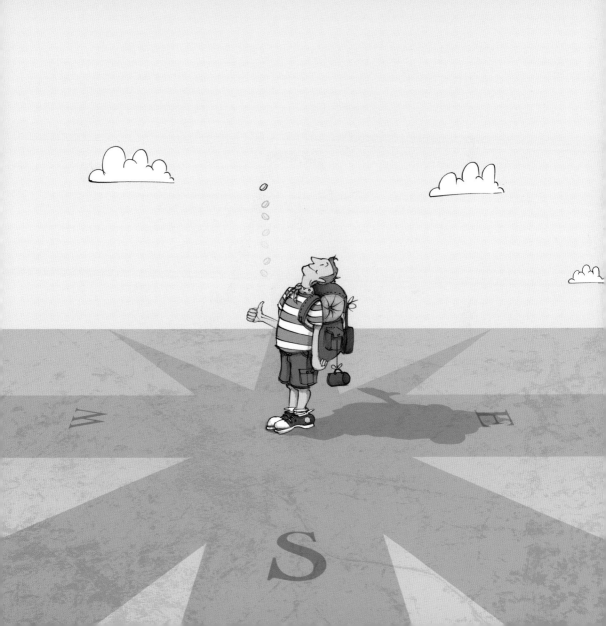

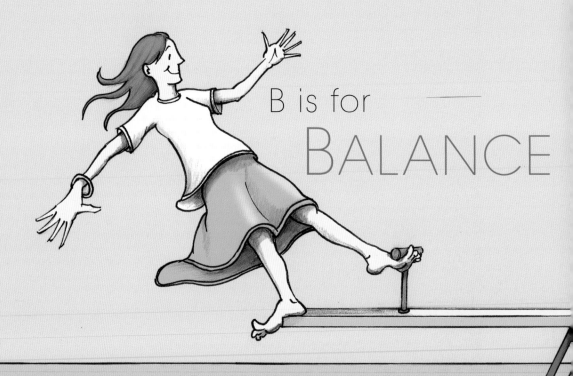

B is for

BALANCE

As humans, we understand things as opposites:
Yin and Yang, good and bad, up and down, day and night.

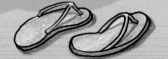

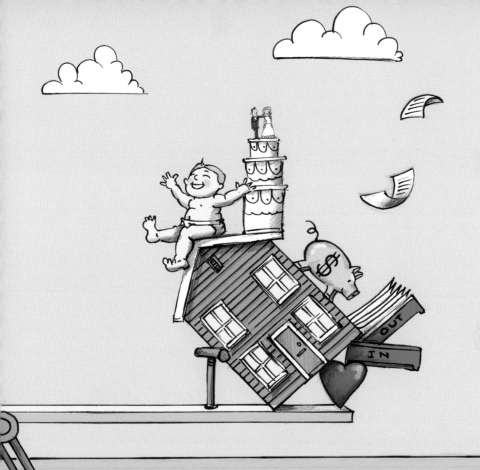

Balance is the tension between opposites: rest and activity, conversation and silence, sociability and solitude, love for another and love for oneself.

Every moment your life is in the balance. Weigh your options.

C is for

Compassion

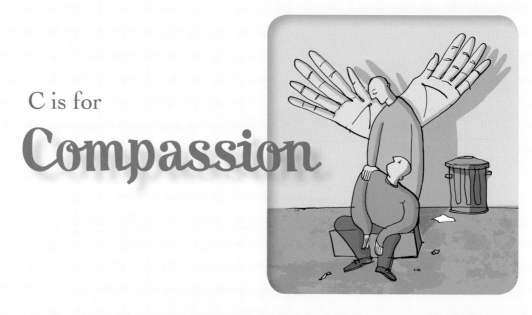

Compassion means to live with love.

It means caring for the sick – and the healthy too.
It means giving to the poor – and to the rich as well.
It means being kind to the needy –
and to those who need for nothing.
Compassion is an equal opportunity emotion.

To make others happy, treat them with compassion.
To make yourself happy, treat others with compassion.

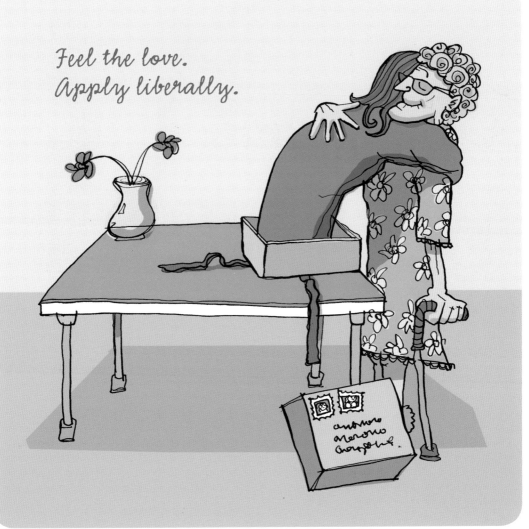

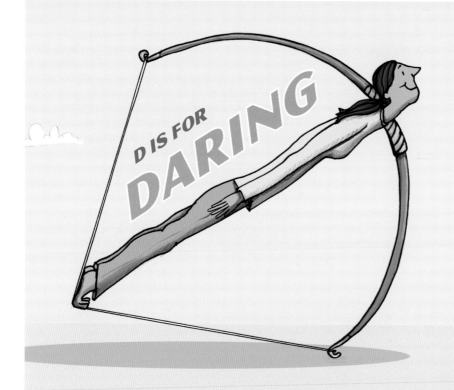

D IS FOR
DARING

Daring is doing. It gets things done.
Every great achievement begins with it.
Every great person first dared to be great.

What will you dare to do today?

DARING IS STEPPING KNOWINGLY INTO THE UNKNOWN.
DARING IS LIVING YOUR LIFE OUT LOUD.
DARING IS WHAT DARING DOES.

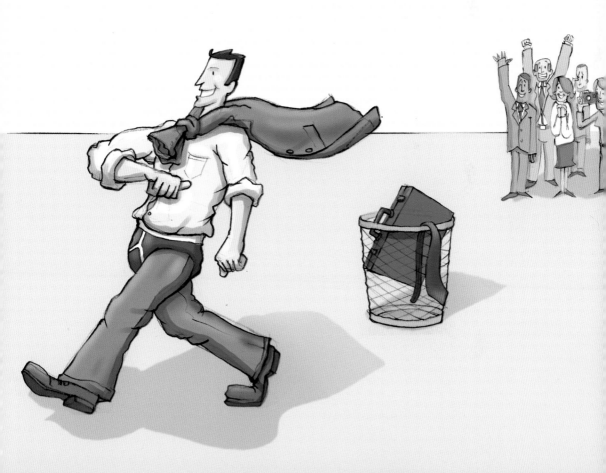

E is for

ENTHUSIASM

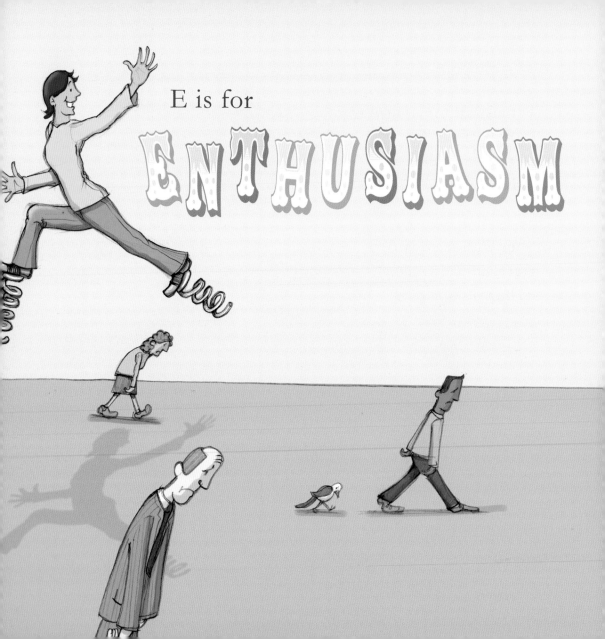

For enthusiasts, life is an adventure, a playground,
a theatre, a movie-set, a laboratory, a love story,
a test track, a roller-coaster, a dance, a gift,
a blessing, a blast, a thrill...

Let your enthusiasm lift you higher.
Wherever it takes you,
it will be the right place.

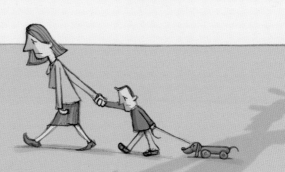

**TO GET ALL YOU CAN FROM LIFE,
PUT ALL YOU CAN INTO IT.**

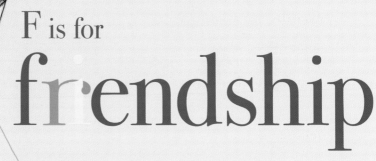

F is for
friendship

Friendship is cheaper than therapy, often deeper.

Feed your friendships and they will sustain you.
Love your friends and you will be loved.
Watch their backs and they will watch yours.

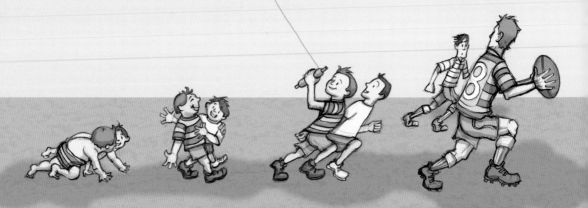

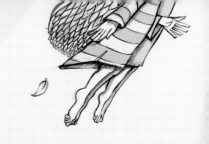

If life's a game, your friends are your team.

Choose them carefully.

Put aside those who bring you down.

Hold on to those who embrace your strengths.

Remember, a good friend is a good listener.

Someone who knows when to say,

'I understand. I am here for you. How can I help?'

In Friendship We Trust.

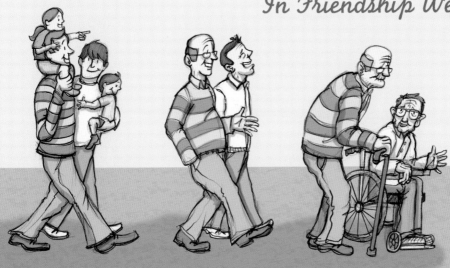

G is for GratituDE

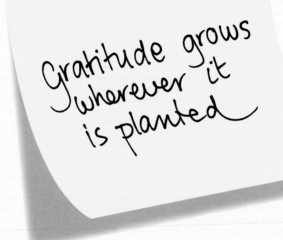

Gratitude grows
wherever it
is planted

Gratitude is more than saying thank you for dinner,
it's saying thank you to life.
When you give thanks, thanks gives back.
So be grateful for what you have,
and you'll have everything you need.

The first sign of greatness is GratituDE.

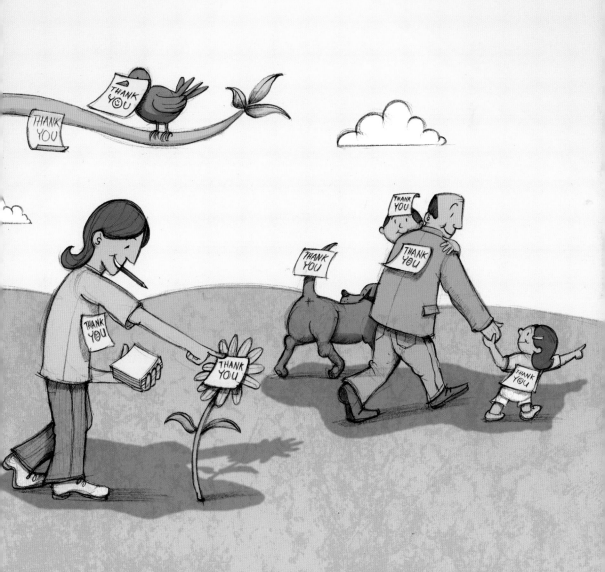

H IS FOR

HOPE

There is one sure thing in life: this too will pass.
No matter your situation, it is certain to change.
However dire things may seem,
there is always a new day, a new way.
Hope helps. Like a rope, it can pull you out of a hole.

THE PROMISE OF BETTER THINGS IS ALWAYS KEP

I is for

Imagination

Think really deeply about something.
Then don't think about it at all.
See what pops up.
Then, once you've had an idea, make it real.
A cake isn't a cake until it's cooked.

Imagine what's possible. Make it happen.

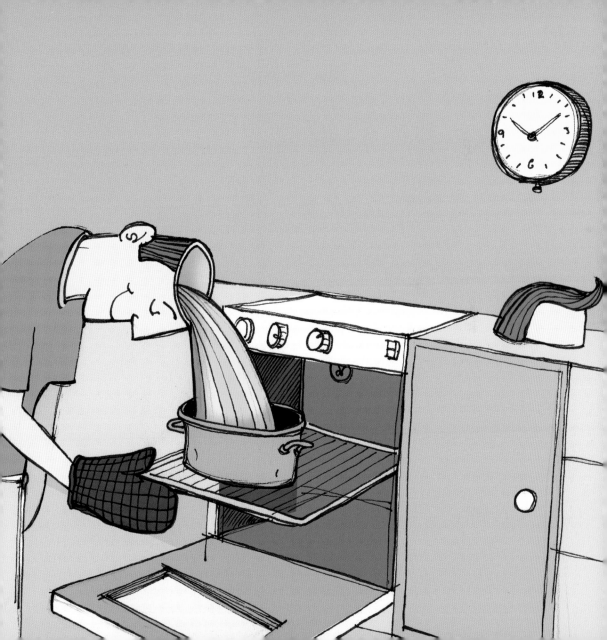

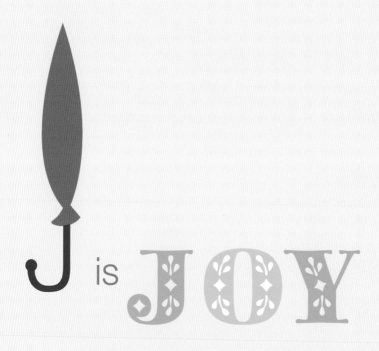

J is **JOY**

Happiness is found deep within.

It comes from our soul – not from external things.

So look inside and feel the joy.

Soon those around you will feel it too.

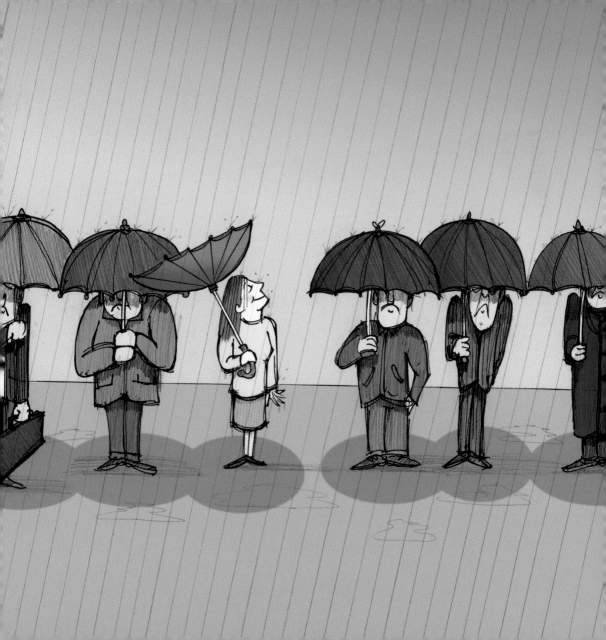

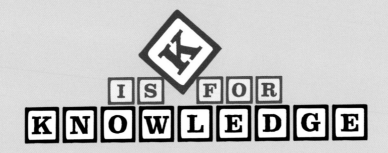

Pass it on.

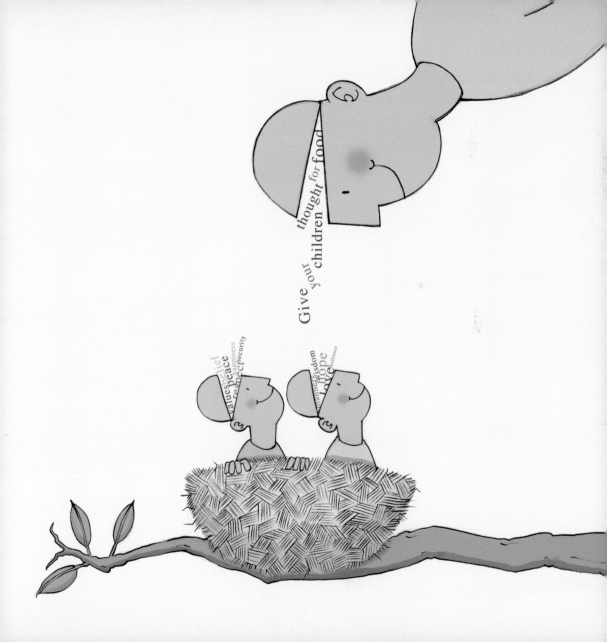

L IS FOR LOVE

In life, we lose our youth, our strength, our influence,
our memory, even our bladder control.

In the end, all we have, and all we will be remembered for, is the
love that we give; not just to one person, but to everyone we meet.
Remember this – and you will be remembered.

What is there to say about love
that has not been said before, except

I love you.

Love is a four letter word. Swear by it.

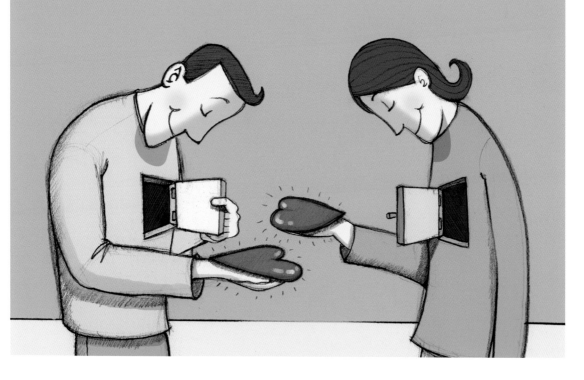

M is for Meditation

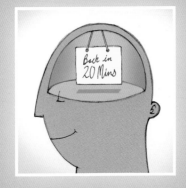

Meditation is a form of medication.
When your soul aches, take a moment.

The more you get into meditation,
the more you get out of it.

So, be mindful – sit in stillness and silence,
watch those thoughts, empty your mind – and live
a full and conscious life.

Because NOW is where it's at.

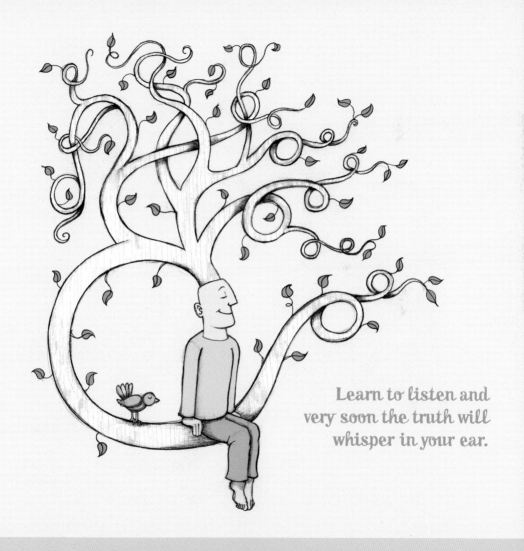

Learn to listen and
very soon the truth will
whisper in your ear.

It really is now or never. Life is fleeting.

Miss the moment and it's gone forever.

To make the most of life, make the most of every moment.

Forget the past, ignore the future, be present to the present. Now.

N is

To be here right now:

Look around. Where are you? How do you feel?

Notice your breathing. The sounds all around you.

Your thoughts as they pass.

See the back of your hand. Look closely. Focus. Observe.

What can you see that you've never seen before?

Be with your hand. Be your hand.

Just be.

BE. HERE. NOW.

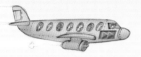

It doesn't matter where you've been.
It doesn't matter where you're going.
It only matters where you're at.

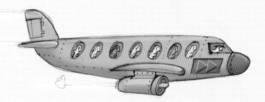

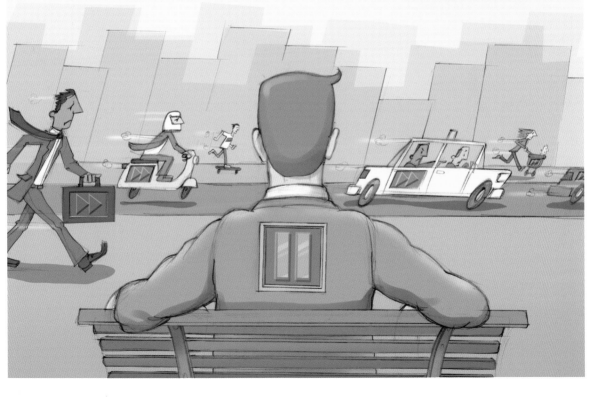

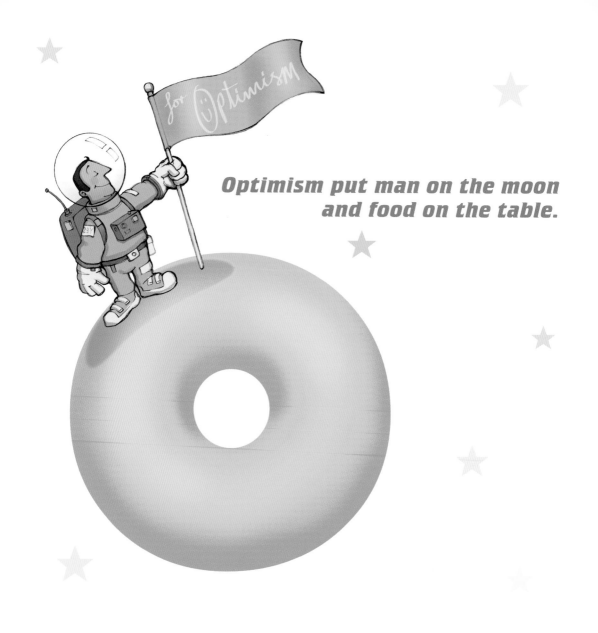

Optimism put man on the moon
and food on the table.

Optimism looks for the best in every situation. The upside of every downside. The yes in every no.

Cultivate it.

Optimism will bring you friendship and success, health and wealth, love and laughter.

It's that kind of word.

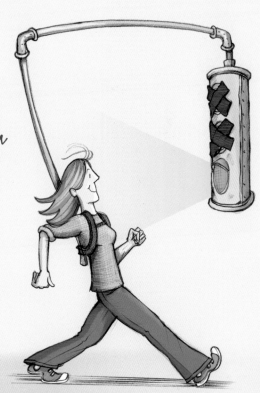

P is for

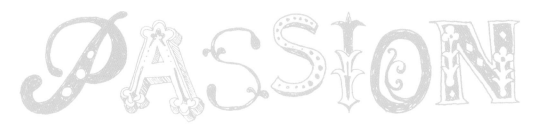

PASSION

Passion has the power to transform your life – to reveal your purpose,

your reason for being, your life's work.

To find out what your passion is, ask yourself 'what would I do

if money was no object?' Paint? Write? Teach? Dance?

Open a vineyard, start a charity, even found a bank?

The trick is to think big, then begin by

taking small, steady steps towards your dream.

Mark Twain said that 'the secret of success is

making your vocation your vacation'.

What would you do if you could do

anything at all?

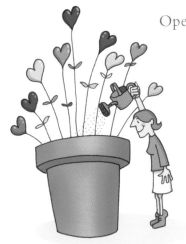

Passion makes anything possible,
everything possible.

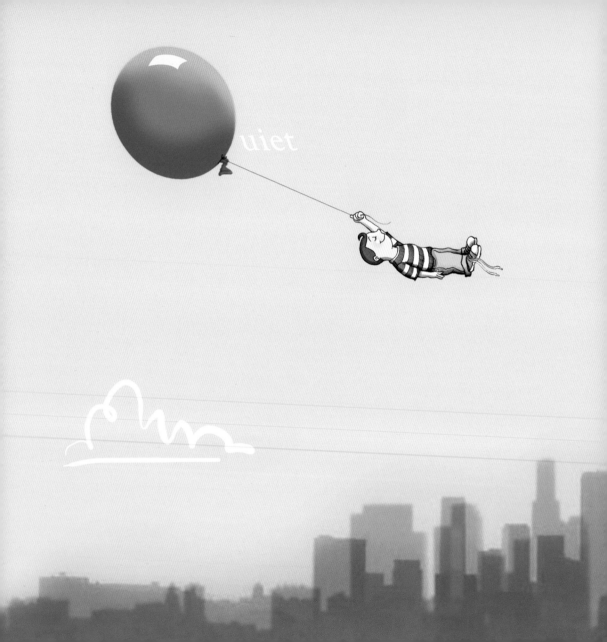

R is for

Reconciliation

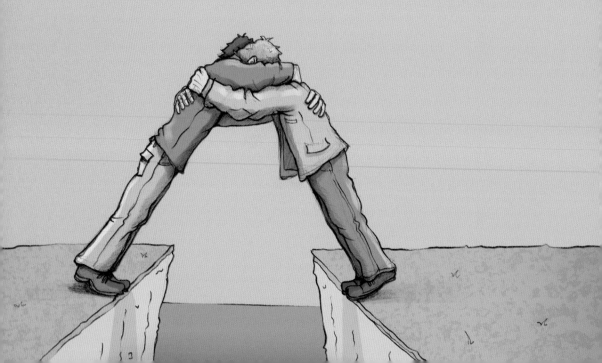

You cannot undo the past.
But you can change the future.
To reconnect with someone,
first forgive yourself.
You're human, you mess up.

Then forgive the other person.
They're human too.

If you do mess up, 'fess up
and apologise.

Saying sorry goes a long way.

Meaning it goes even further.

Remember: the sooner you can laugh about it,
the sooner you can laugh about it together.

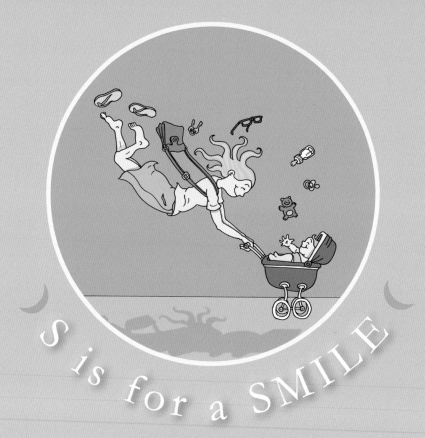

S is for a SMILE

Unleash the power of a smile.
Smile at strangers. Smile at trees.
Smile at misfortune.
Smile at yourself in the mirror in the morning.
Smile just for the sake of it.
Soon fortune will smile back at you.

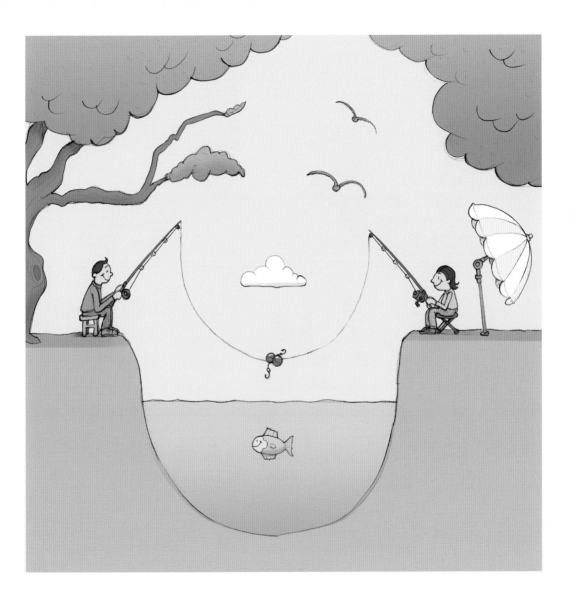

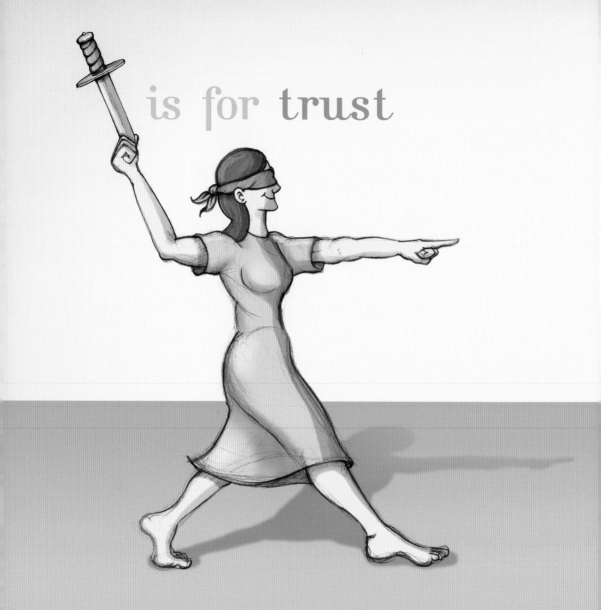

is for trust

Trust is the bedrock of love,

the mattress of marriage,

the cradle of childhood,

the foundation of friendship.

Trust in the truth and,

the truth is,

you'll be trusted.

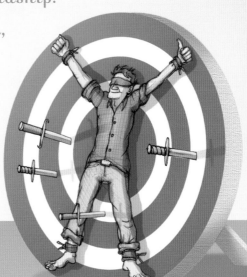

U is the Universe

When things are looking down, look up.
Sometimes realising our cosmic
insignificance can put our
troubles into perspective.

Have faith, trust in Fate, be free.
The Universe is there to support you.
Climb on board.

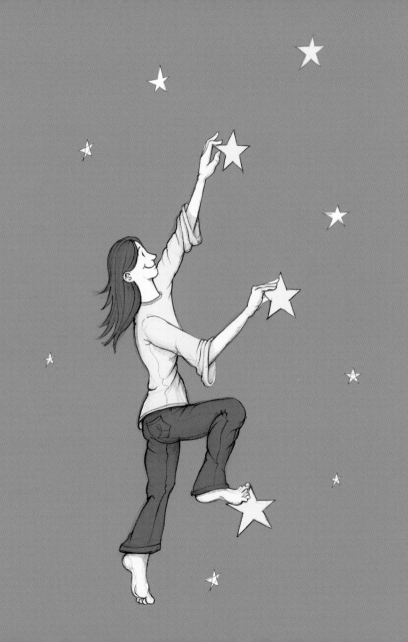

V is for VISION

To understand what your vision is, ask the Big Questions.

Who am I? What are my values? What do I want to teach, to pass on?

These are the beginnings of a vision.

One day you will ask yourself, 'What kind of life have I lived?'

WHAT WILL YOUR ANSWER BE?

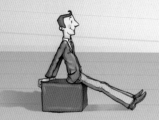

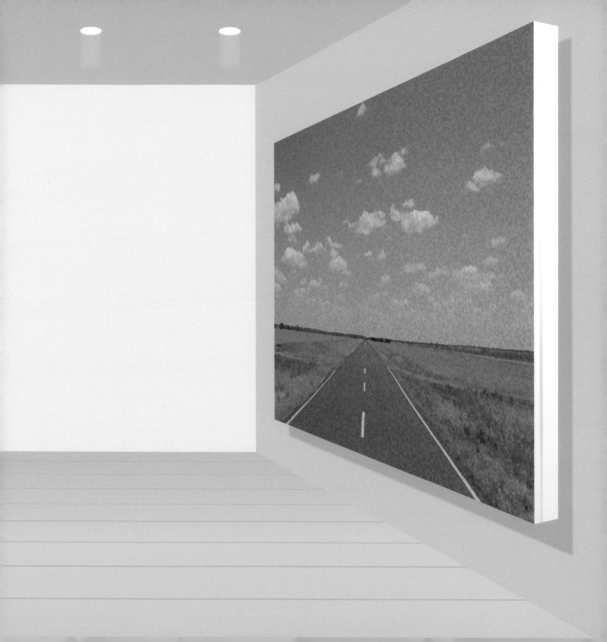

W is Wisdom

Knowing isn't wisdom.

Knowing yourself is.

There is more wisdom in contentment

– accepting life and everything in it –

than is contained in all the libraries of the world.

Your soul is a book – study it carefully.

Share what you've learned.

If you go out looking for wisdom,

it won't know where to find you.

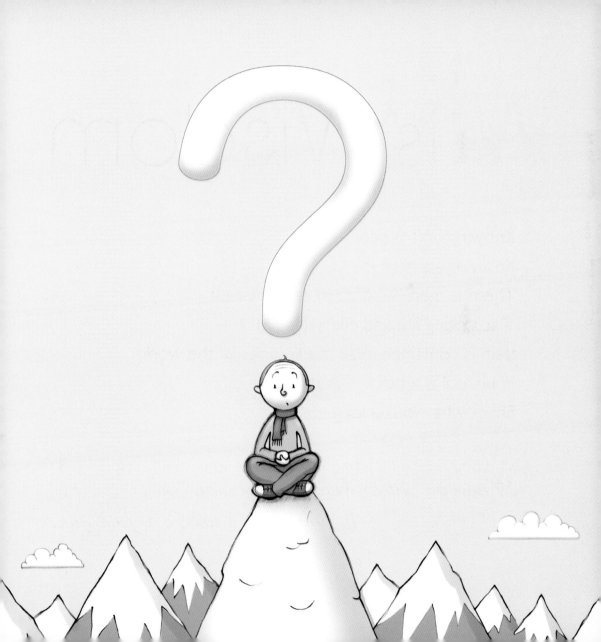

X IS A KISS

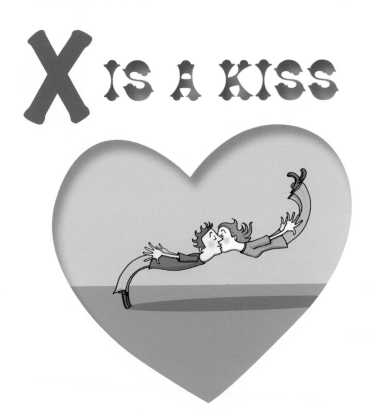

A kiss shows love and intimacy, tenderness and desire.
It can say hello or goodbye, good luck or good riddance, adoration
or adulation. It can say things that can otherwise never
be said, speaking without words, communicating without sound.

What will you say with a kiss today?
And who will you say it to?

X X X X

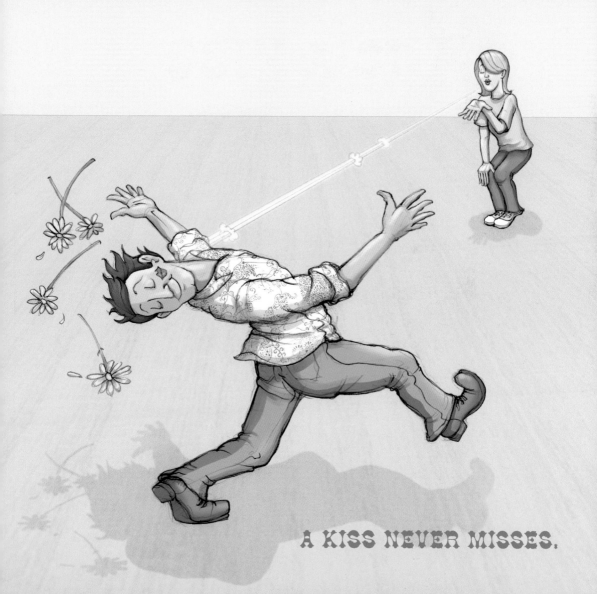

A KISS NEVER MISSES.

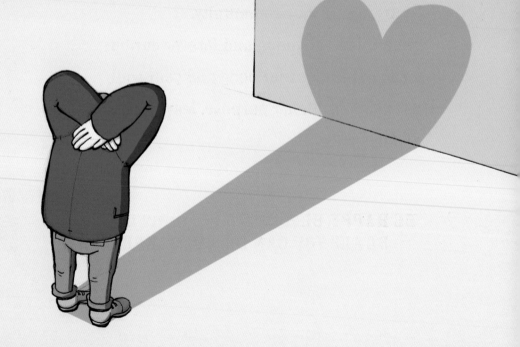

To live a full and satisfying life,

think with your heart, be loyal to your dreams,

engage your emotions, respect your relationships,

defy your fears, pursue your passions, find your flow,

express your energy, enjoy the moment,

contribute to your community,

remain forever young and forever curious,

feed your mind, your body and your soul,

answer your higher purpose, leave a legacy,

and live with love.

BE HAPPY. **BE HONEST.** BE HOPEFUL.
BE ALL YOU CAN BE. **BE YOURSELF.**

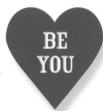

ZEN IS OUR NORMAL CONDITION.
IT IS A STATE OF BEING.

OF SILENCE. PEACEFULNESS.
WAKEFULNESS. MINDFULNESS.

RIGHT VIEW.
RIGHT INTENTION.
RIGHT SPEECH.
RIGHT ACTION.

ZEN IS THE PLACE TO BE.

BALANCE YOUR BEING AND
YOUR LIFE WILL BE IN BALANCE.

LIVE RIGHT AND
EVERYTHING WILL BE ALL RIGHT.

SIT IN STILLNESS AND SILENCE.

TURN YOUR EYE INWARD.

ZEN IS OUR NORMAL CONDITION.
IT IS A STATE OF BEING.
OF SILENCE. PEACEFULNESS
WAKEFULNESS. MINDFULNE...
RIGHT VIEW.
RIGHT INTENTION.
RIGHT SPEECH.
RIGHT ACTION.

ZEN IS THE PLACE TO BE.

BALANCE YOUR BEING AND
YOUR LIFE WILL BE IN BA...
LIVE RIGHT AND
EVERYTHING WILL BE ALL RIG...
SIT IN STILLNESS AND SILENCE.
TURN YOUR EYE INWARD.

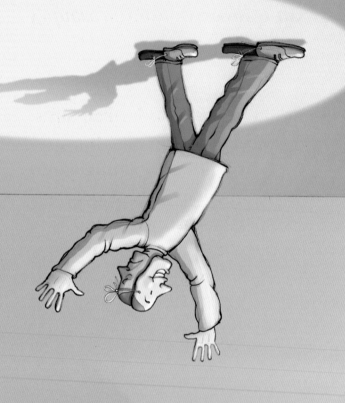

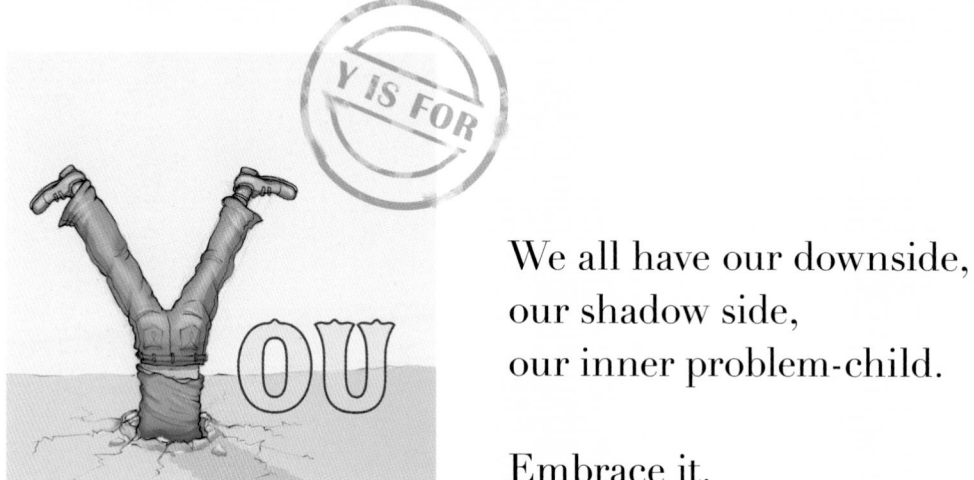

We all have our downside,
our shadow side,
our inner problem-child.

Embrace it.

Admitting our weaknesses is the first step
in regaining our strength.
Confronting our demons is the first act
in reclaiming our soul.
Shining light on our darkness
is the beginning of enlightenment.

Vulnere viresco — through my wound I grow strong.

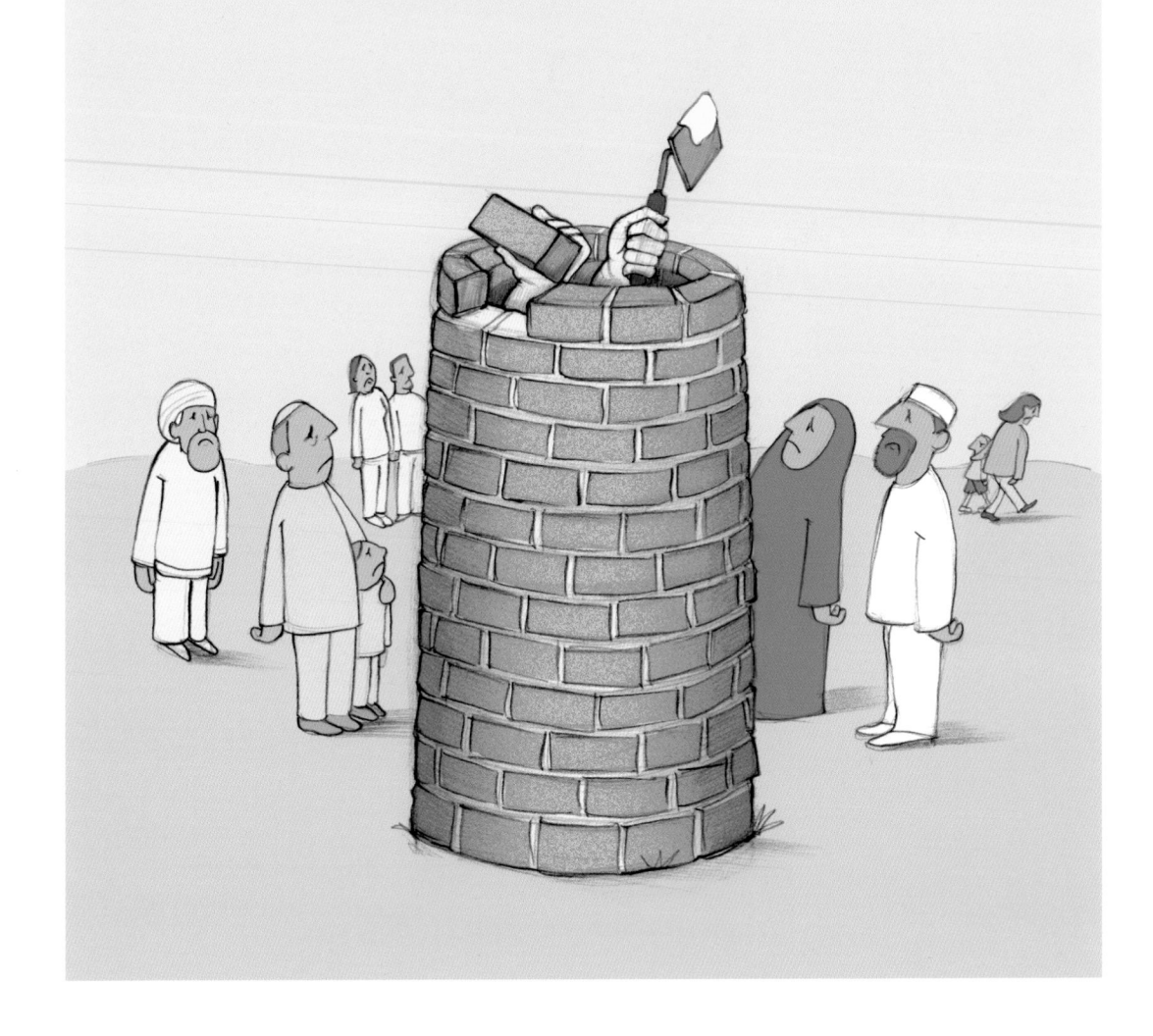

X is for Xenophobia

[zen-*uh*-foe**-be-*uh*]**

Xenophobia is an ugly word.
Xeno means foreigner. Phobia is fear.

Together they mean racism, bigotry,
intolerance, injustice.

Yet, if we embrace the differences in this world,
the world looks different.

More interesting, more rewarding, more –

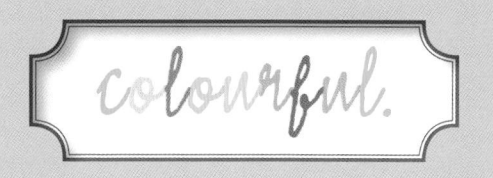

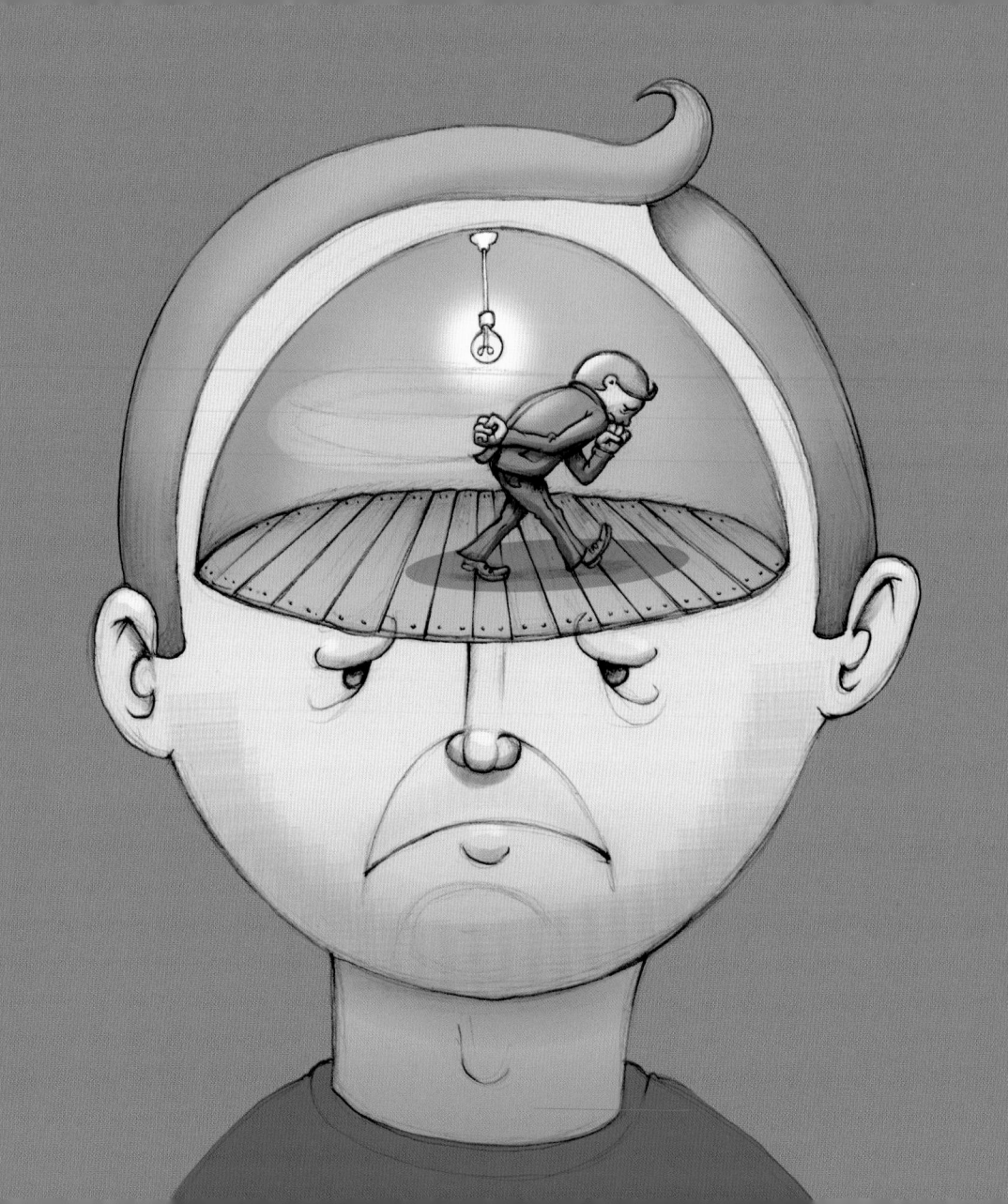

W is for WORRY

Worry is your brain in too much of a hurry.

To get on top of it, get over yourself.

Helicopter over your thoughts.

Observe their patterns and themes.

Let them go. They're not facts, and not fixed.

Like clouds, they will pass.

Let them go.

Let them be.

Just be.

Thoughts.

Coming and going.

Nothing to worry about.

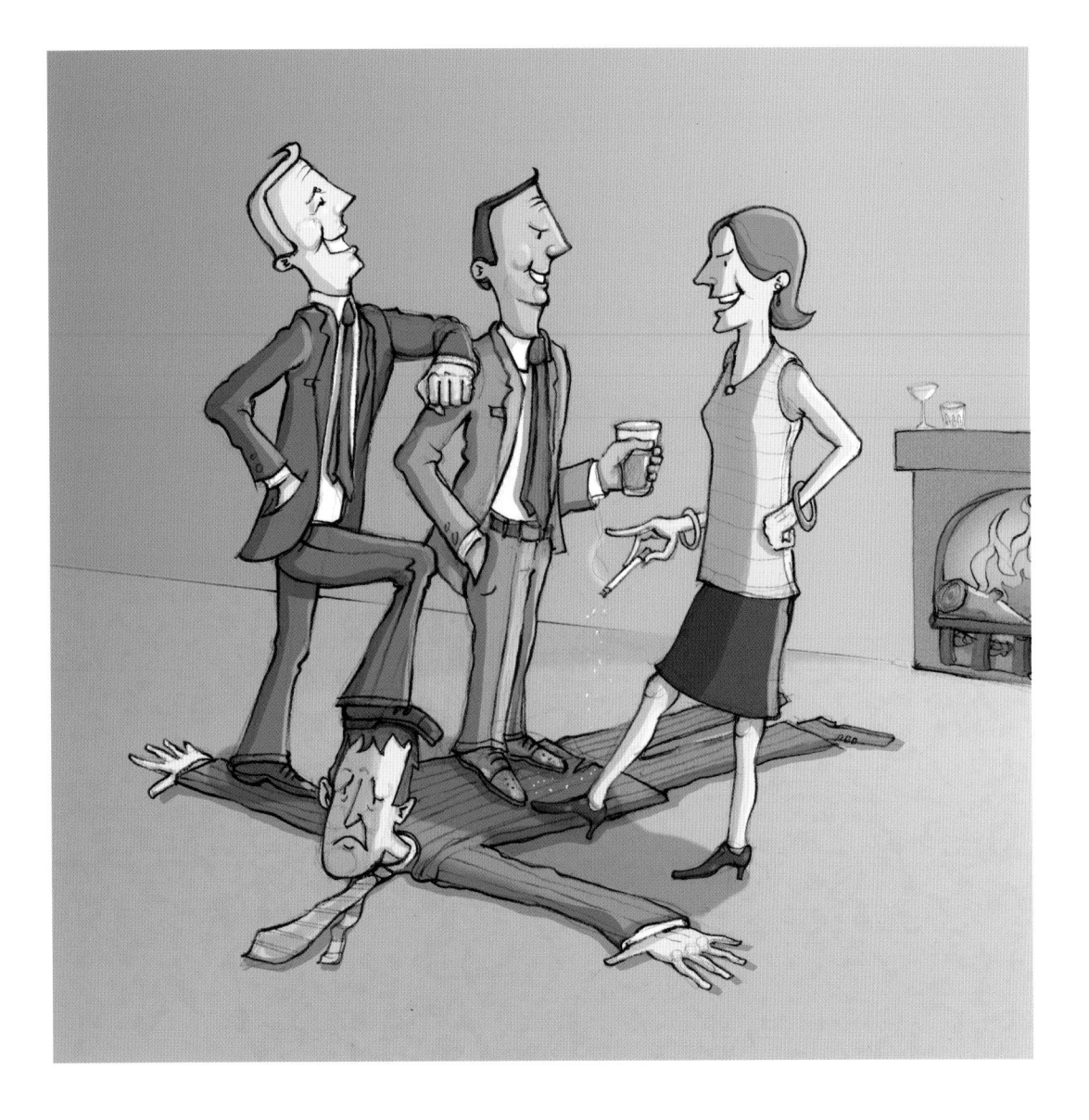

V is for

VICTIMHOOD

We can't control what happens in life —
but we can control the way we respond.
This means eliminating self-pity, blame and victimhood.

Bad things happen to good people — but being the victim
keeps you in the past, robs you of the present, steals your future.

The remedy? Accept what has happened.
Don't blame yourself. Move forward.

**ASK NOT WHAT THE WORLD HAS DONE TO YOU,
BUT WHAT YOU CAN DO FOR THE WORLD.**

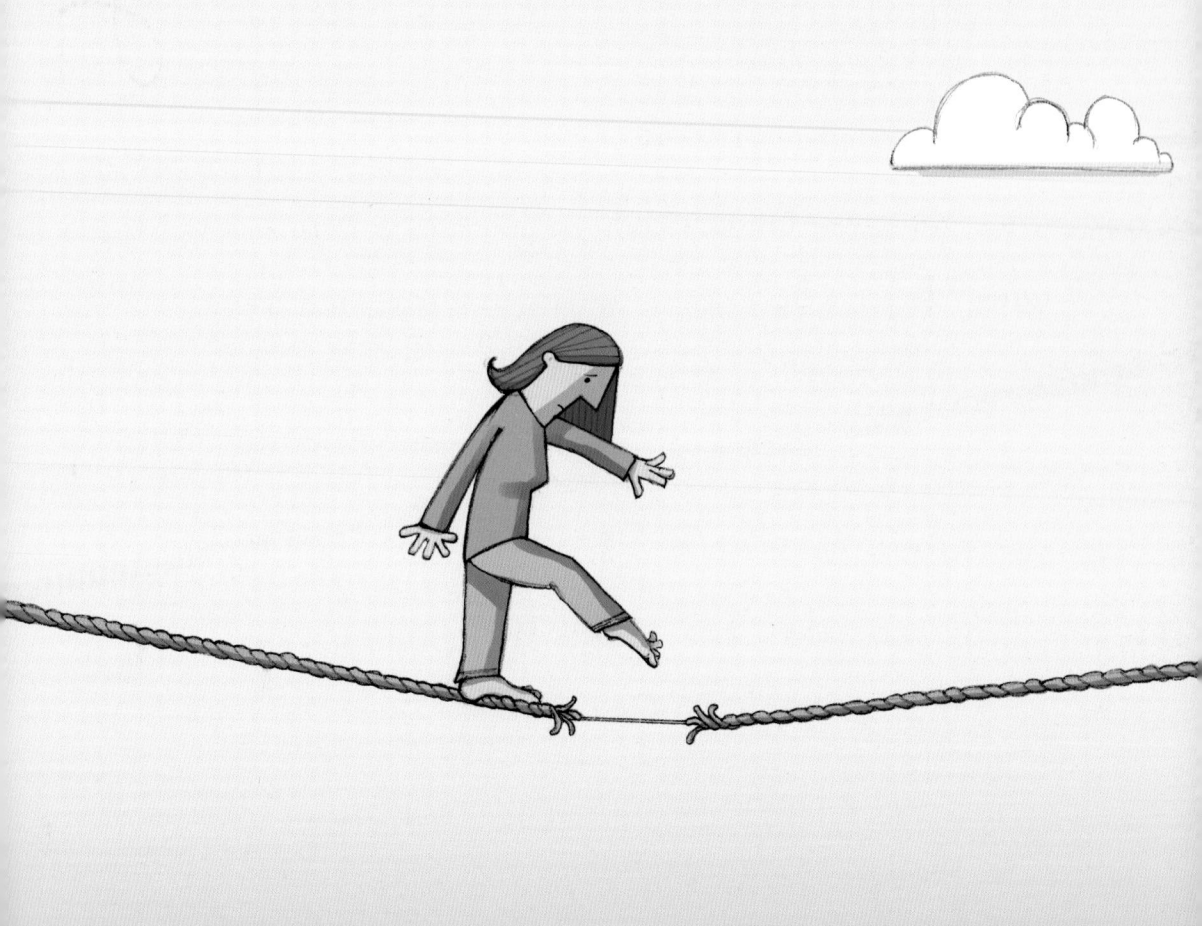

U is for Uncertainty

One thing is certain in life— nothing is certain.
The best way to deal with uncertainty is one step at a time.
You can never know which way things will fall— but if
your life is in balance, you will land on your feet.

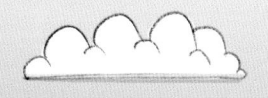

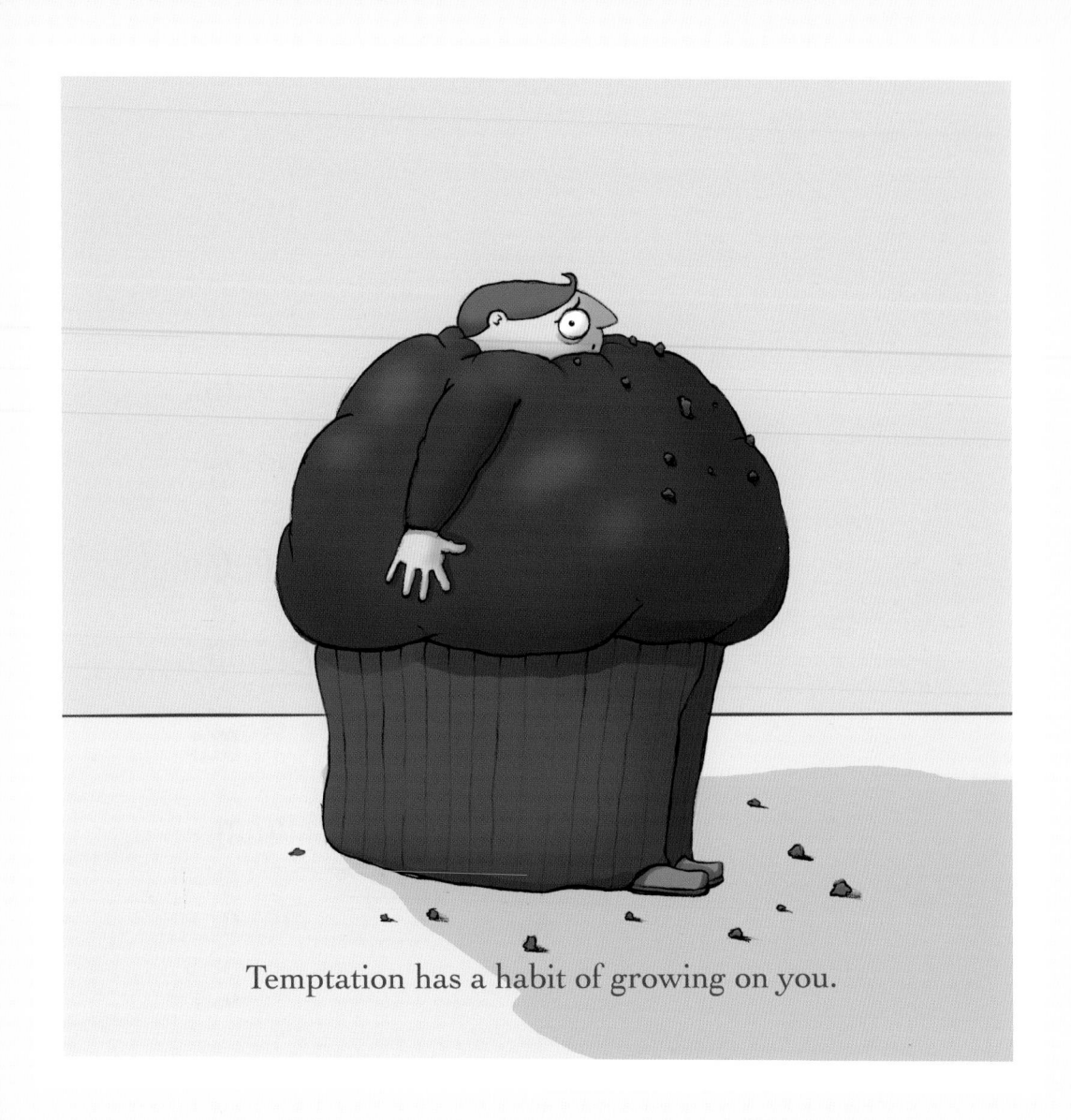

Temptation has a habit of growing on you.

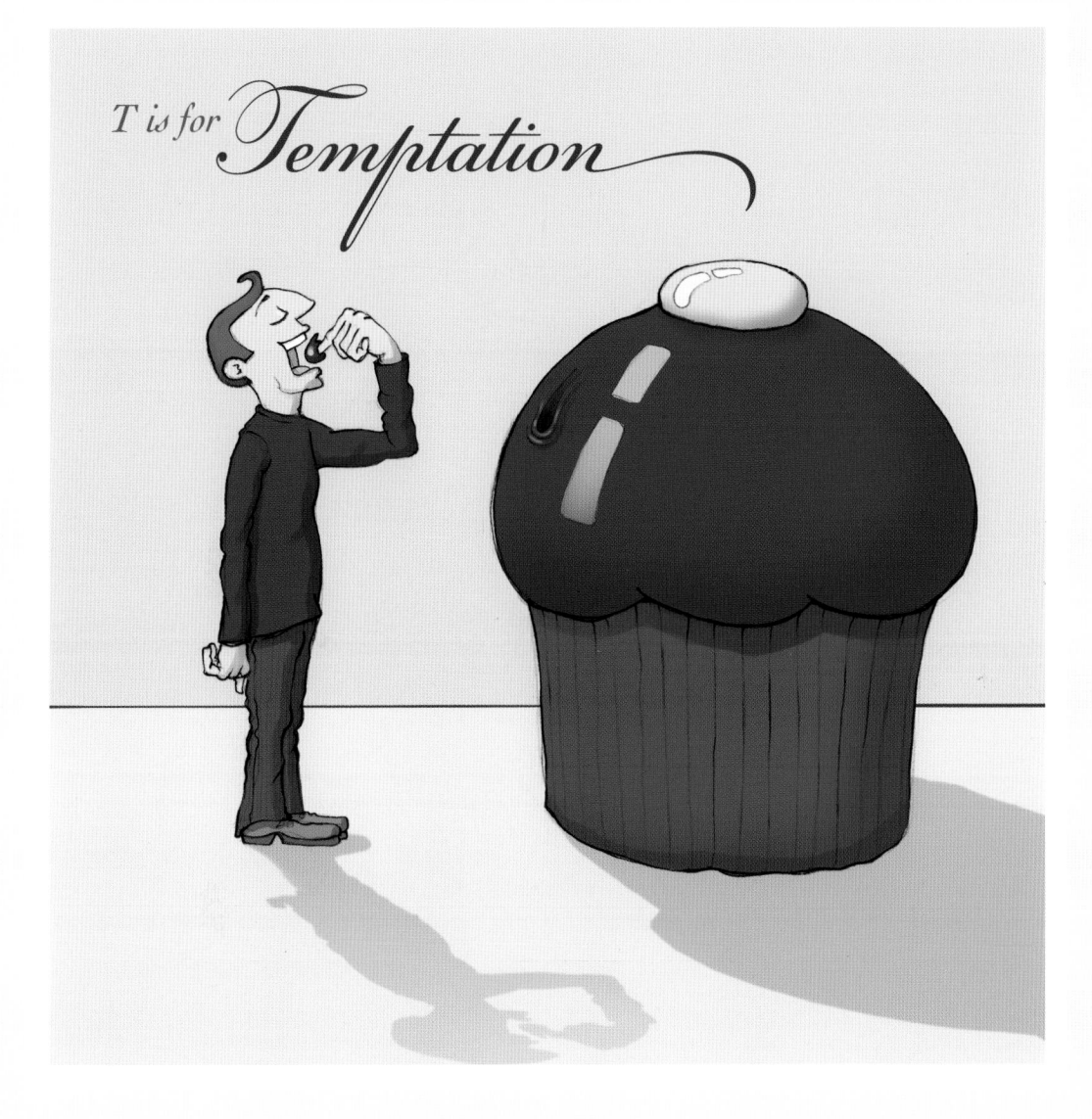

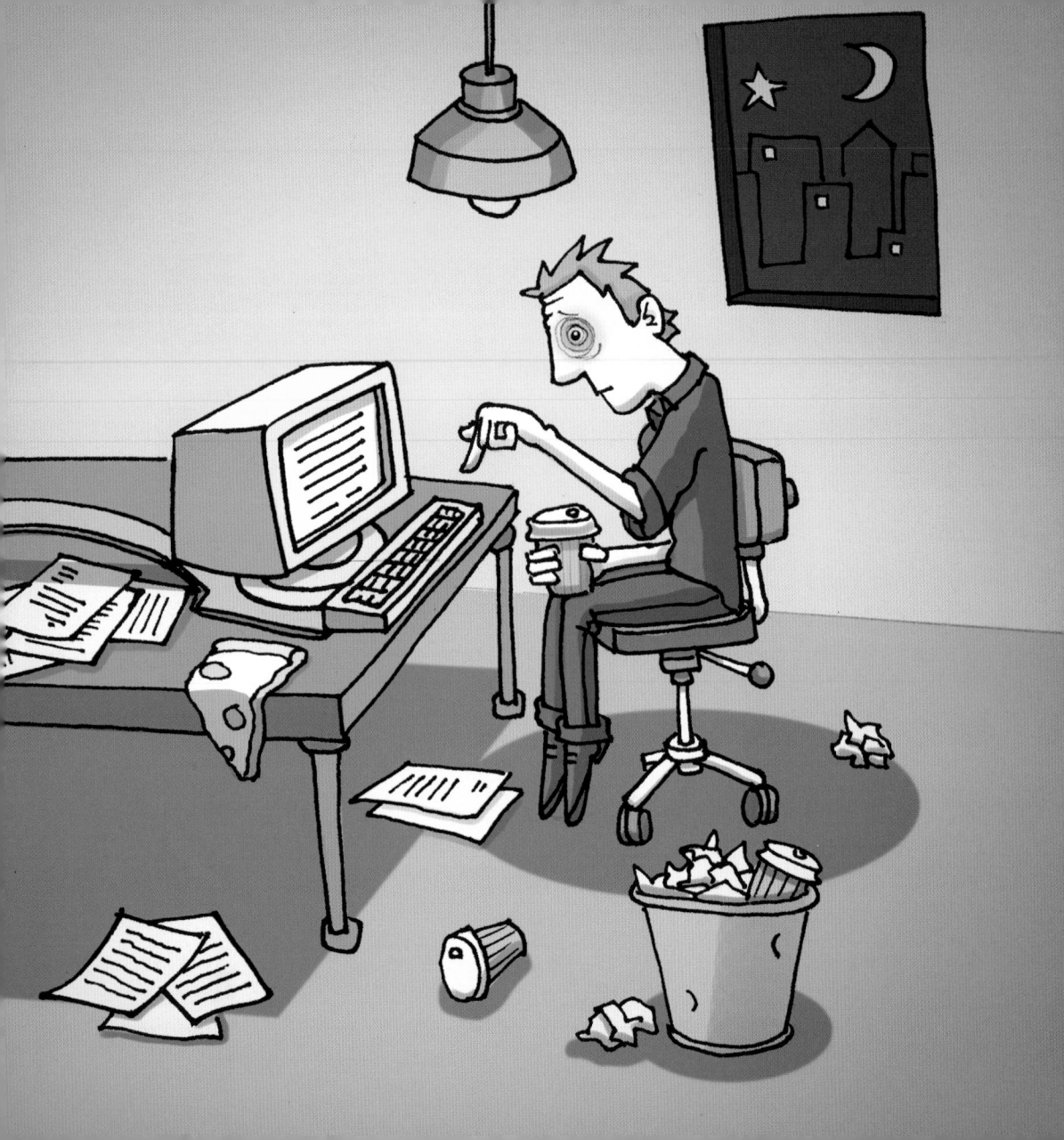

S is for STRESS

Insomnia. Heartache. Anxiety. Depression.
The cost of stress is never worth the salary that demands it.
When designing your work life, make sure that your life works.

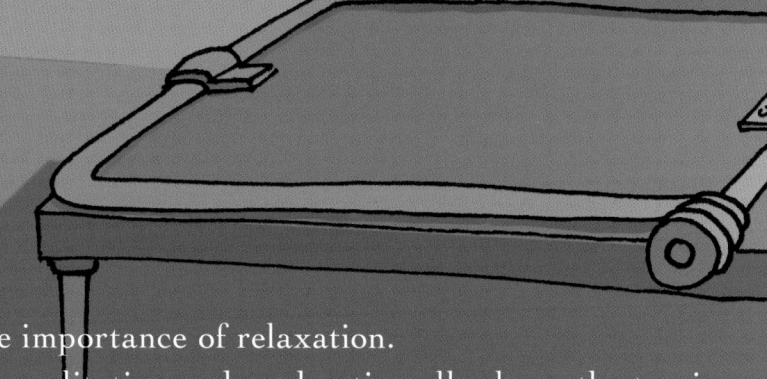

Stress the importance of relaxation.
Exercise, meditation and moderation all release the tension.
Drink, drugs, and junk food don't.

So, unwind your mind.
A little stress is healthy, too much can kill you.
Deal with it before you snap.

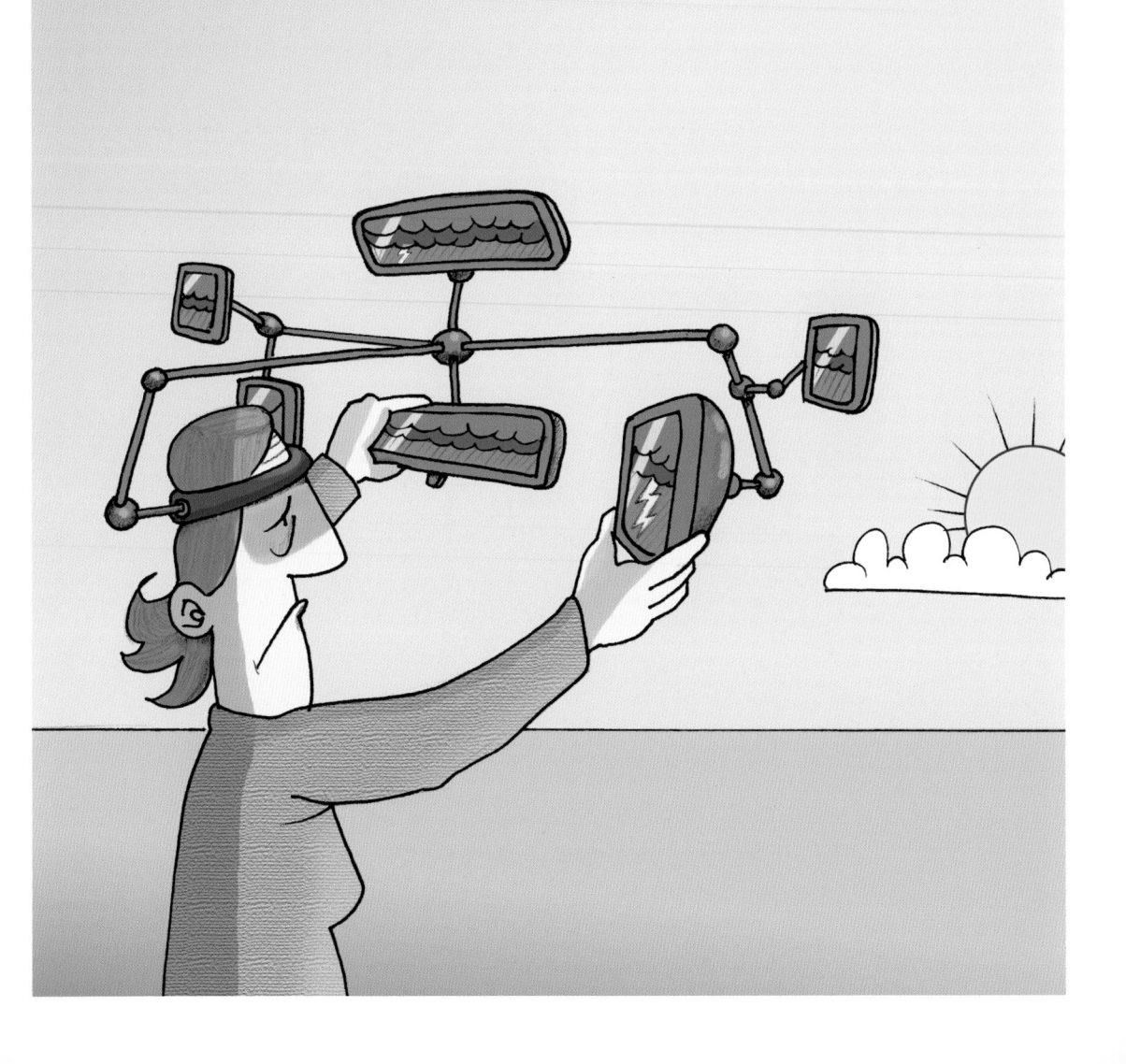

R IS FOR REGRET

Stuff happens.
But it doesn't need to keep happening.
Regret keeps us living in the past,
dragging us backwards, holding us back.
To get over it, get into the moment.
Empty your mind, let go of your thoughts, just be.

Be forgiving. Be loving. Be grateful.

LET THE PAST BE PAST.

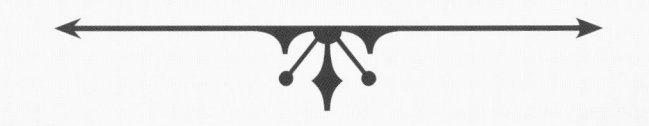

Sometimes, the only thing we have to beat
is our desire to give up.
Overcome this and you can overcome anything.

Never give up on your dreams.
Never give up on you.
Never give up.

Never.
Ever.

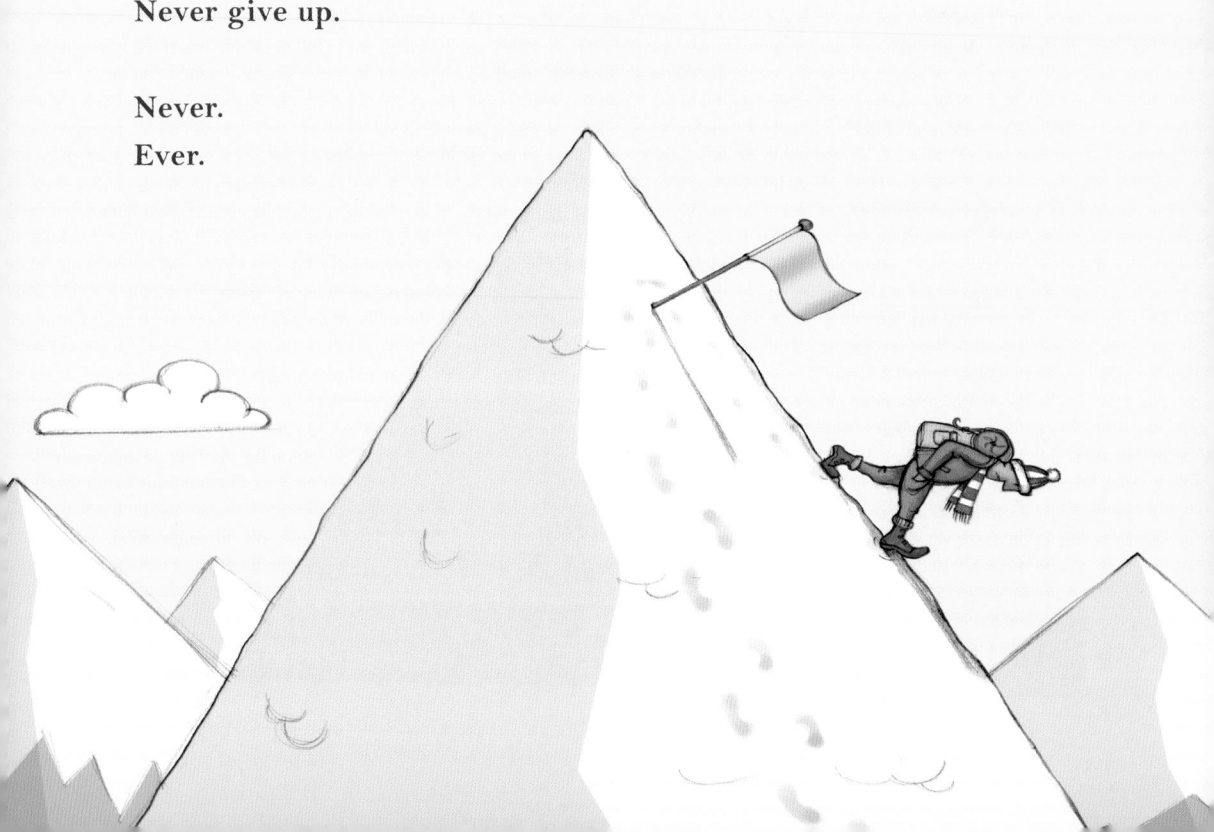

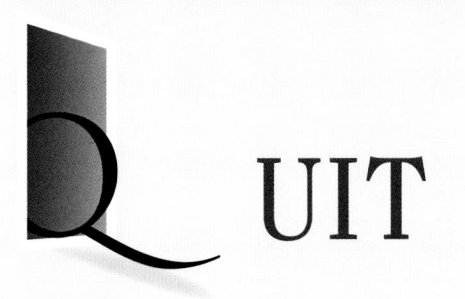 UIT

To give up is to give in to the voice that says 'it doesn't matter'.

It does. You know it does.

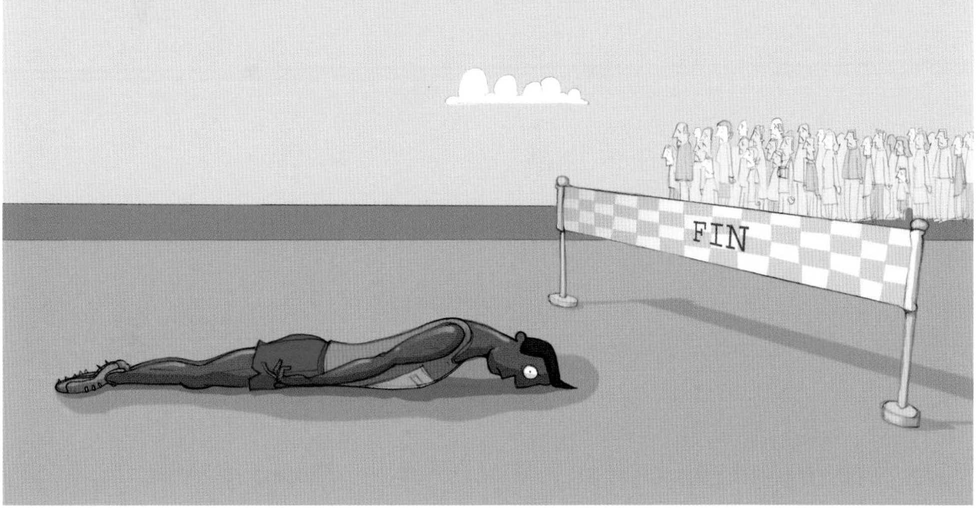

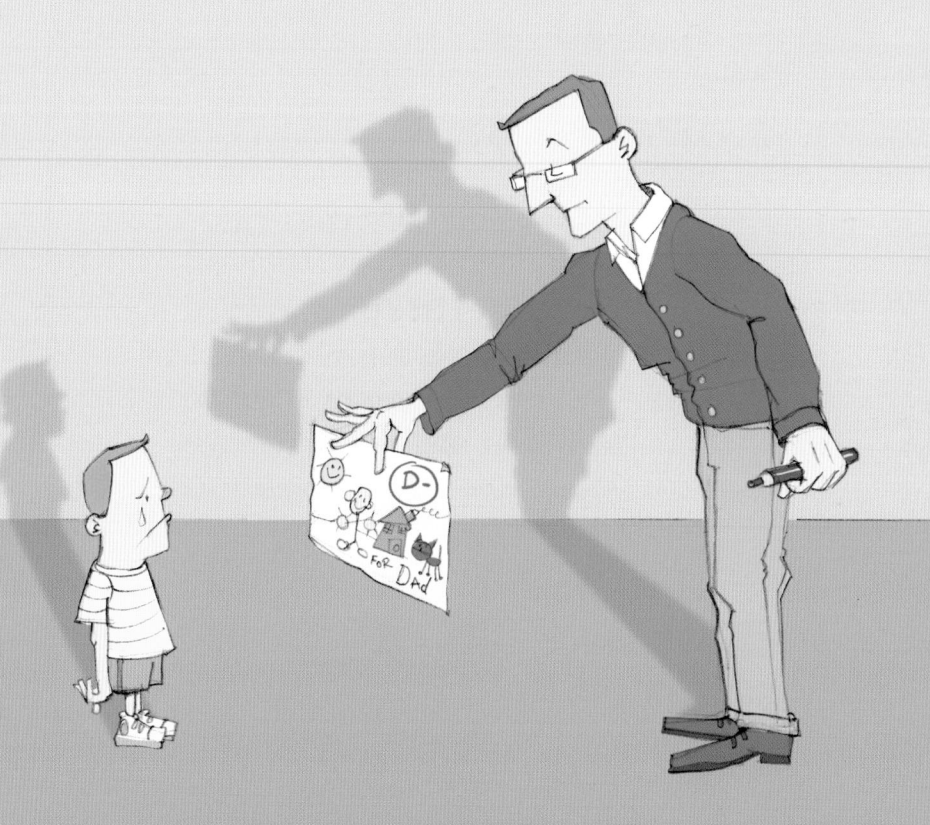

Perfectionism is always a mistake.

P is for Perfectionism

Trying to get something exactly right
is the best way of getting it wrong.

Perfection is a kind of paralysis.

The tighter you hold onto something the more it will hold you back.

Often the best way to improve something is to let it go.

So do the best that you possibly can, finish it, and relax.

It will be better than you think. It might even be perfect.

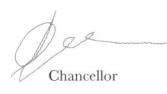

Chancellor

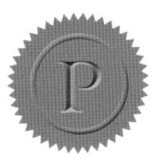

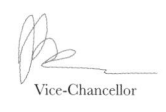

Vice-Chancellor

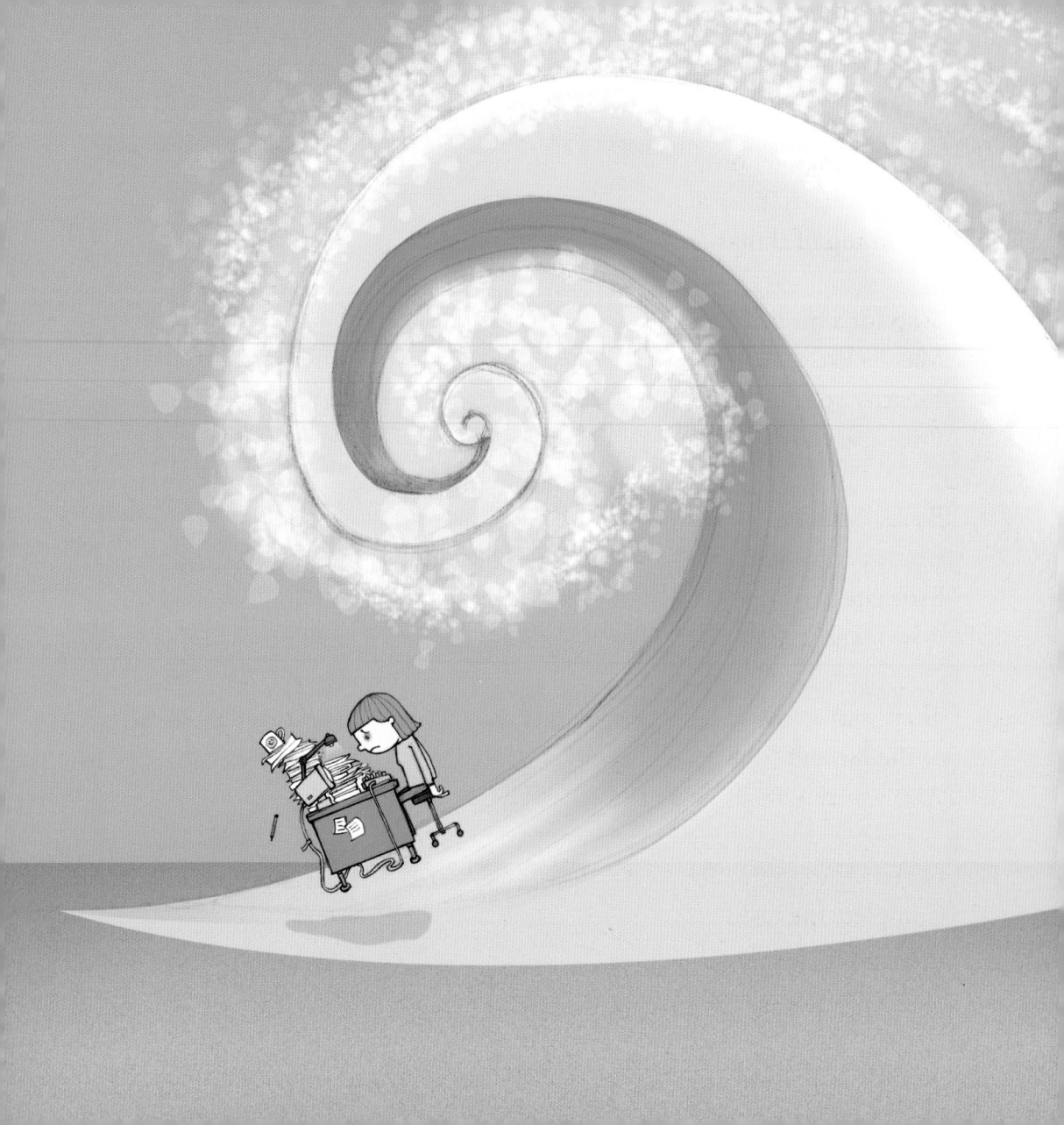

When things get on
top of you, it's time to
get on top of things.

Stop for a moment.
Make a list.
Identify your priorities.
Prioritise your priorities.

Be realistic about
what is achievable.
Estimate the time
it will take. Double it.

Then start at the top
of the list and work
your way down.

Do one thing at a time.
Complete the task.
Cross it off.
Start another.

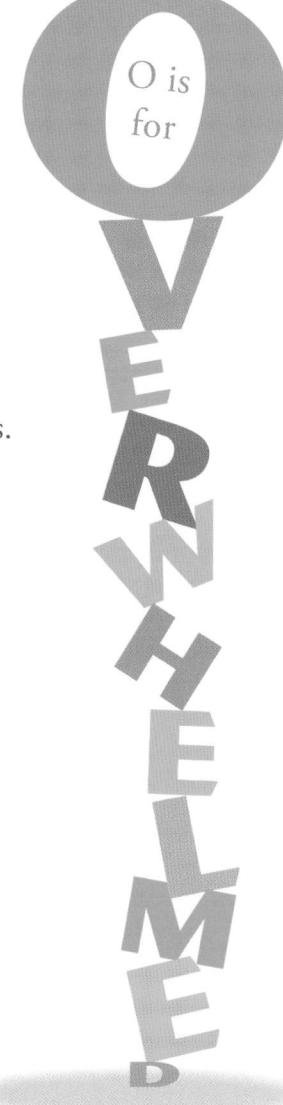

O is for

OVERWHELMED

Remember:

ONE.
THING.
AT.
A.
TIME.

If you start thinking
about all the work that
needs to be done, stop.
Think only about the
work that you're doing.
And do it.

That way, the work
that needs to be done,
gets done.

NEGATIVITY

Life looks the way you look at it.
A positive point of view sees a brighter future.
A negative perspective paints a bleaker universe.
Always remember that your outlook will be your outcome.

A few small changes can make a huge difference.

For instance, try saying yes to every question

you're asked (within reason).

You'll discover new places, meet new people,

and live a happier and richer life.

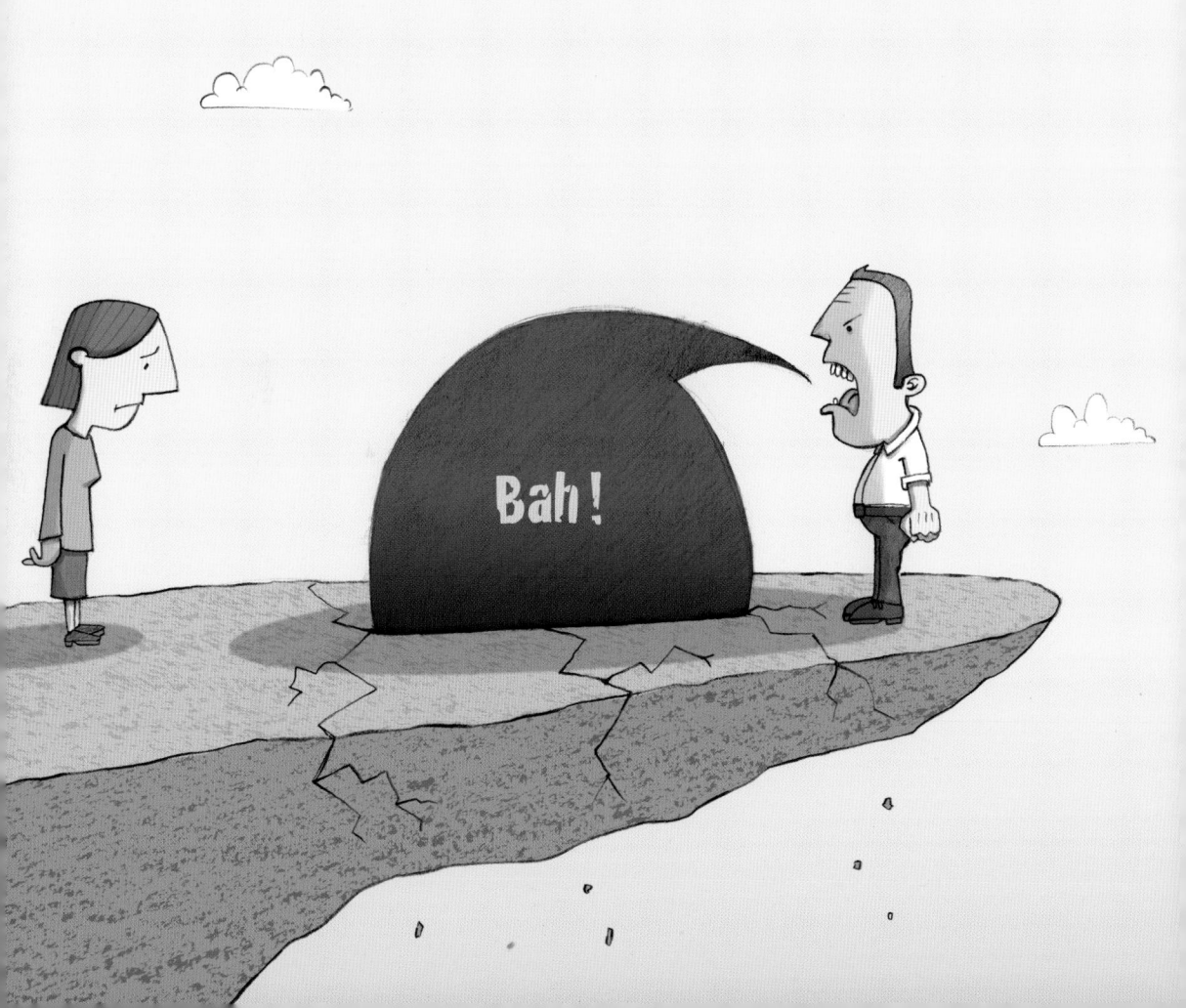

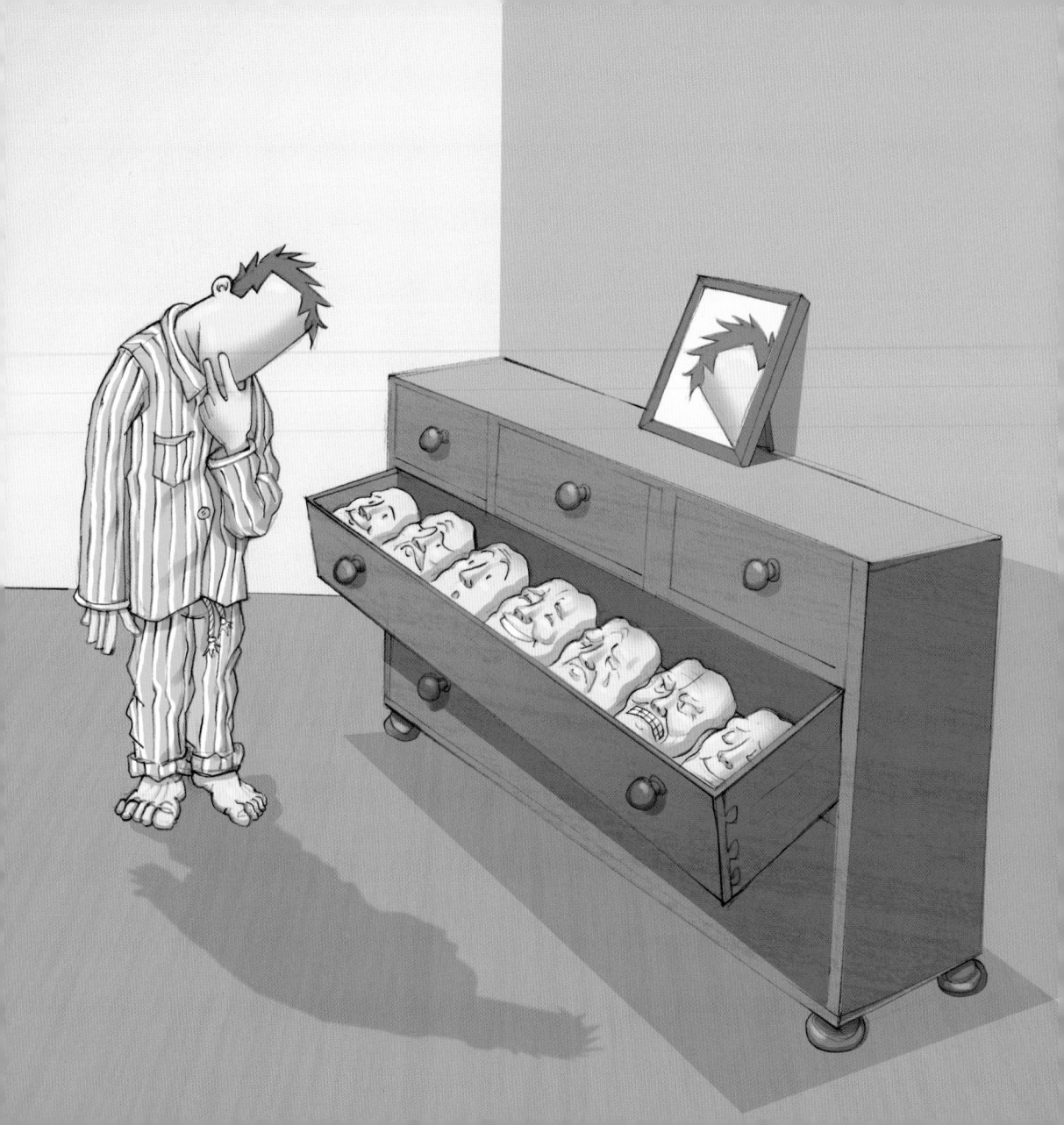

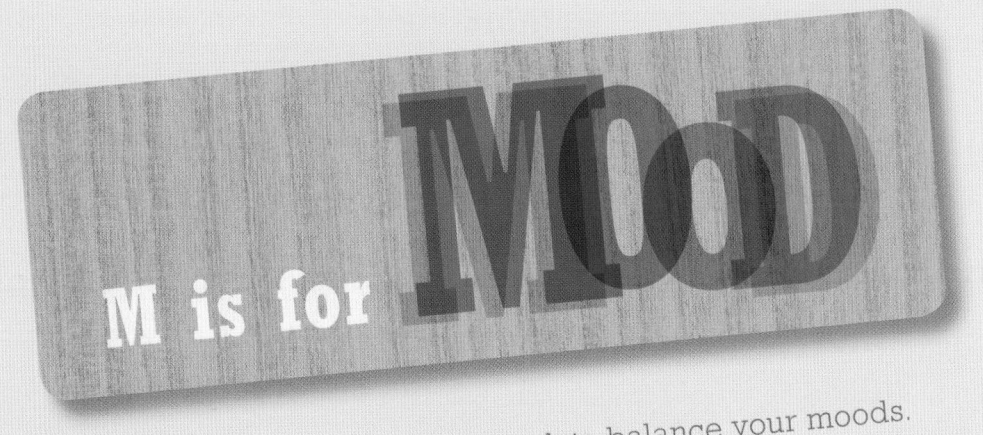

M is for MOOD

If your life is out of balance, seek to balance your moods.
Many things can cause them to swing.
Drink. Drugs. Diet. Stress.
To find balance, go back to basics.
Bring your body and your mind down to earth.
Sleep well, eat healthily, exercise.
And choose your thoughts carefully.

**Where your thoughts go,
your moods will follow...**

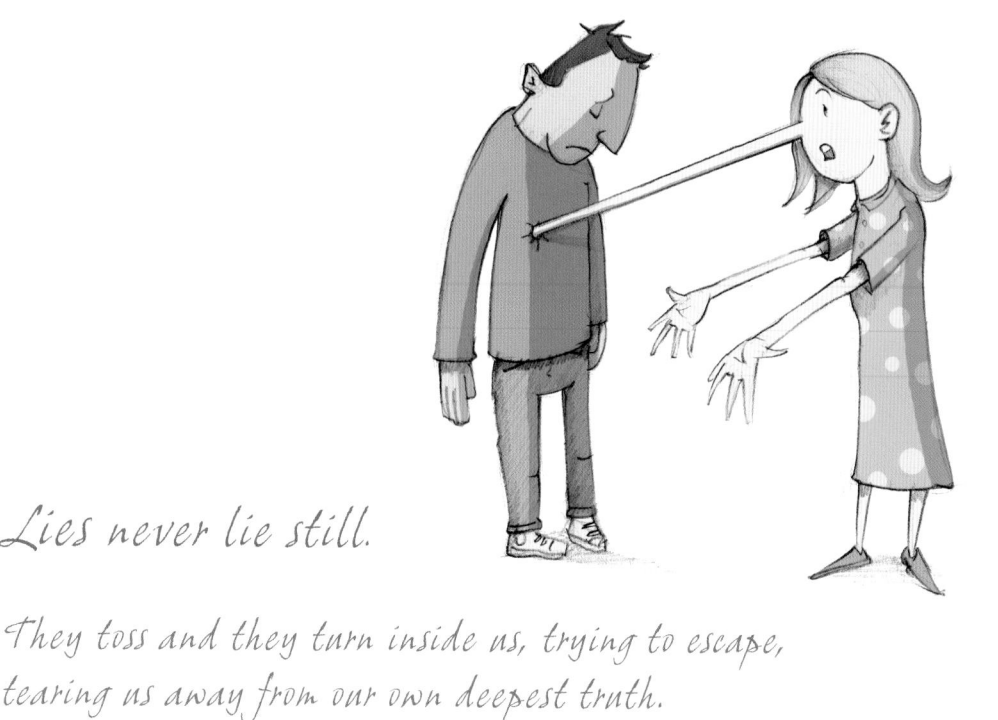

Lies never lie still.

They toss and they turn inside us, trying to escape,
tearing us away from our own deepest truth.
If you lie, ask yourself 'why?'

Lies often cover our deepest fears: of being discovered,
found out, unmasked; of being seen for who we really are.
To be all you can be — tell the truth.
It might hurt at first to admit it, but it will truly set you free.

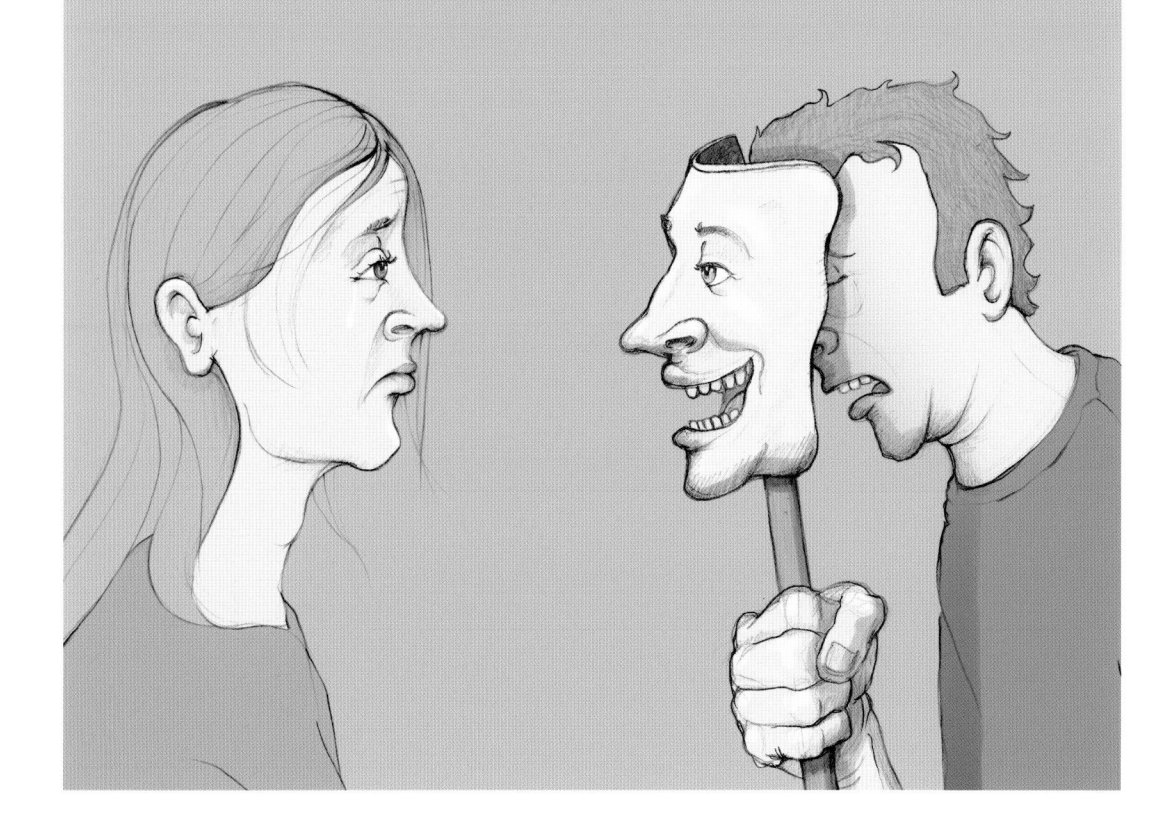

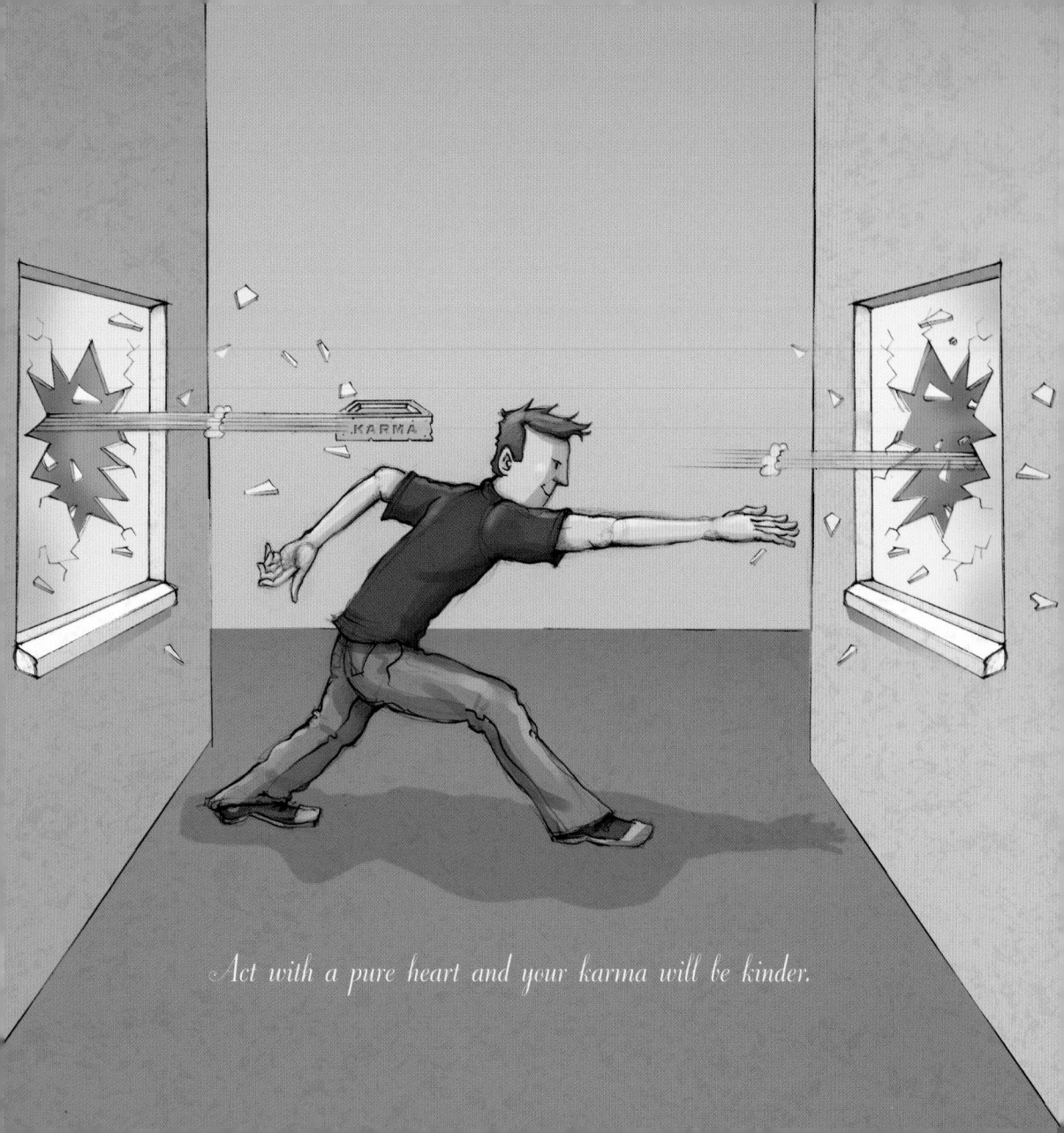

Act with a pure heart and your karma will be kinder.

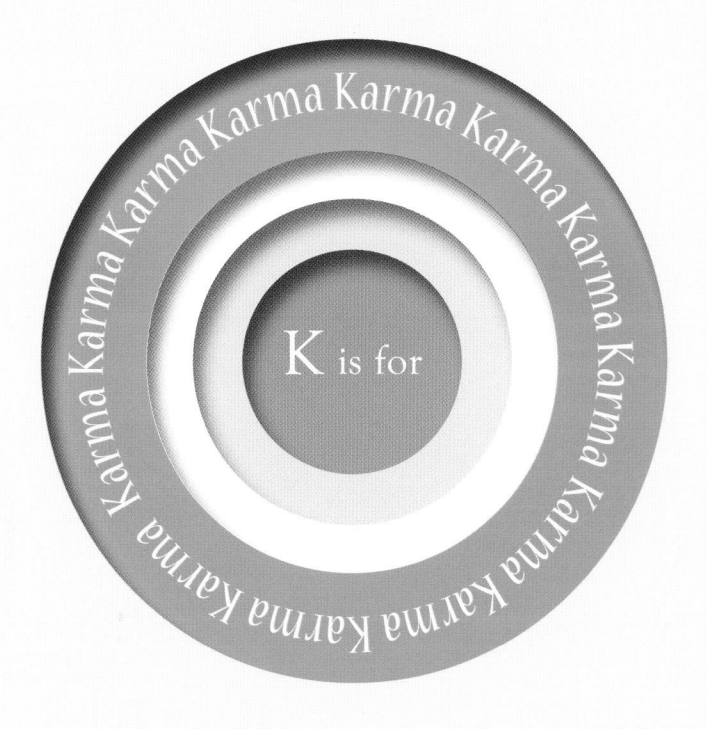

K is for

Karma Karma Karma Karma Karma Karma Karma Karma Karma Karma Karma Karma Karma Karma Karma Karma

Karma is Sanskrit for 'deed' or 'act'.
It is the law of cause and effect, part of the
Buddhist cycle of past, present and future.
Whether your karma is good or bad
depends on your intentions.

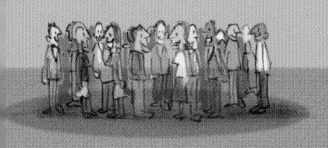

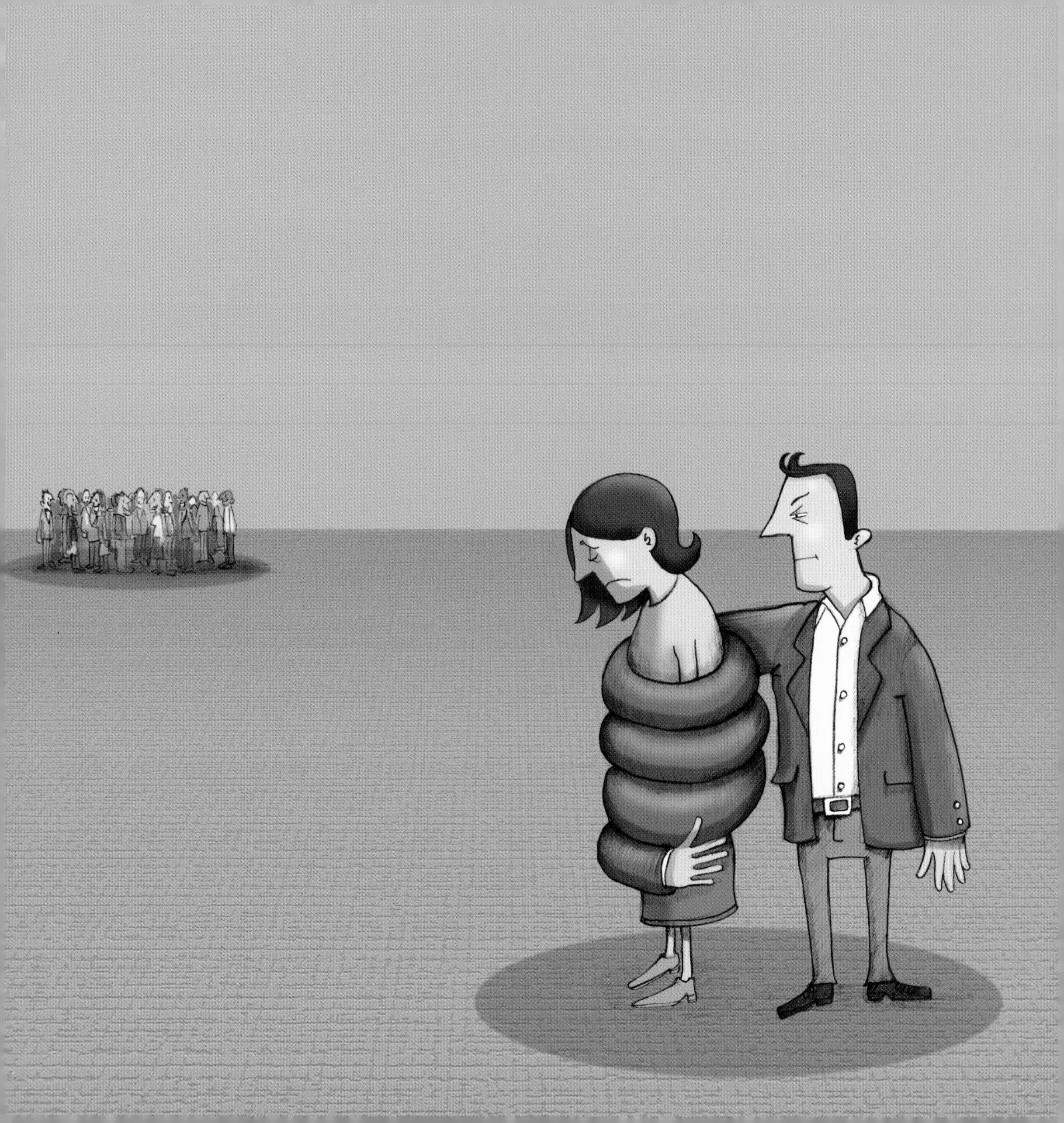

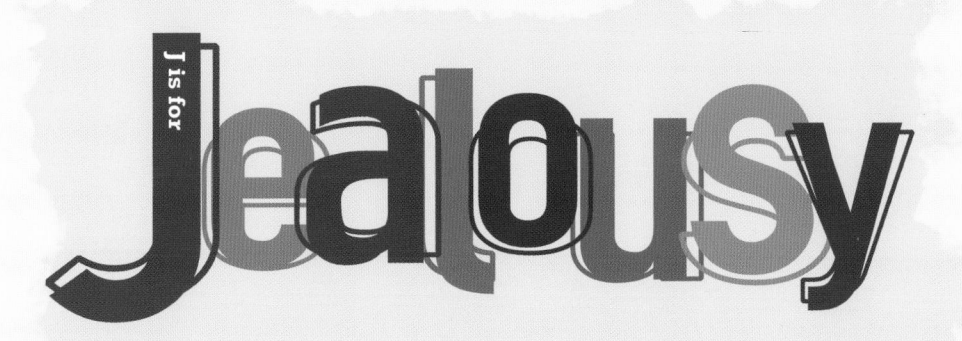

J is for **Jealousy**

Jealousy kills the love it seeks to protect.

It can remind you of who and why you love –

but it brings with it pain and anxiety and heartbreak.

To save your relationship, lose your jealousy.

This isn't easy. It takes time and effort.

Truthfulness and trust.

Patience and perseverance.

Reality checks and reassurance.

It's a labour of love.

Jealousy is a snake; cut off its head.

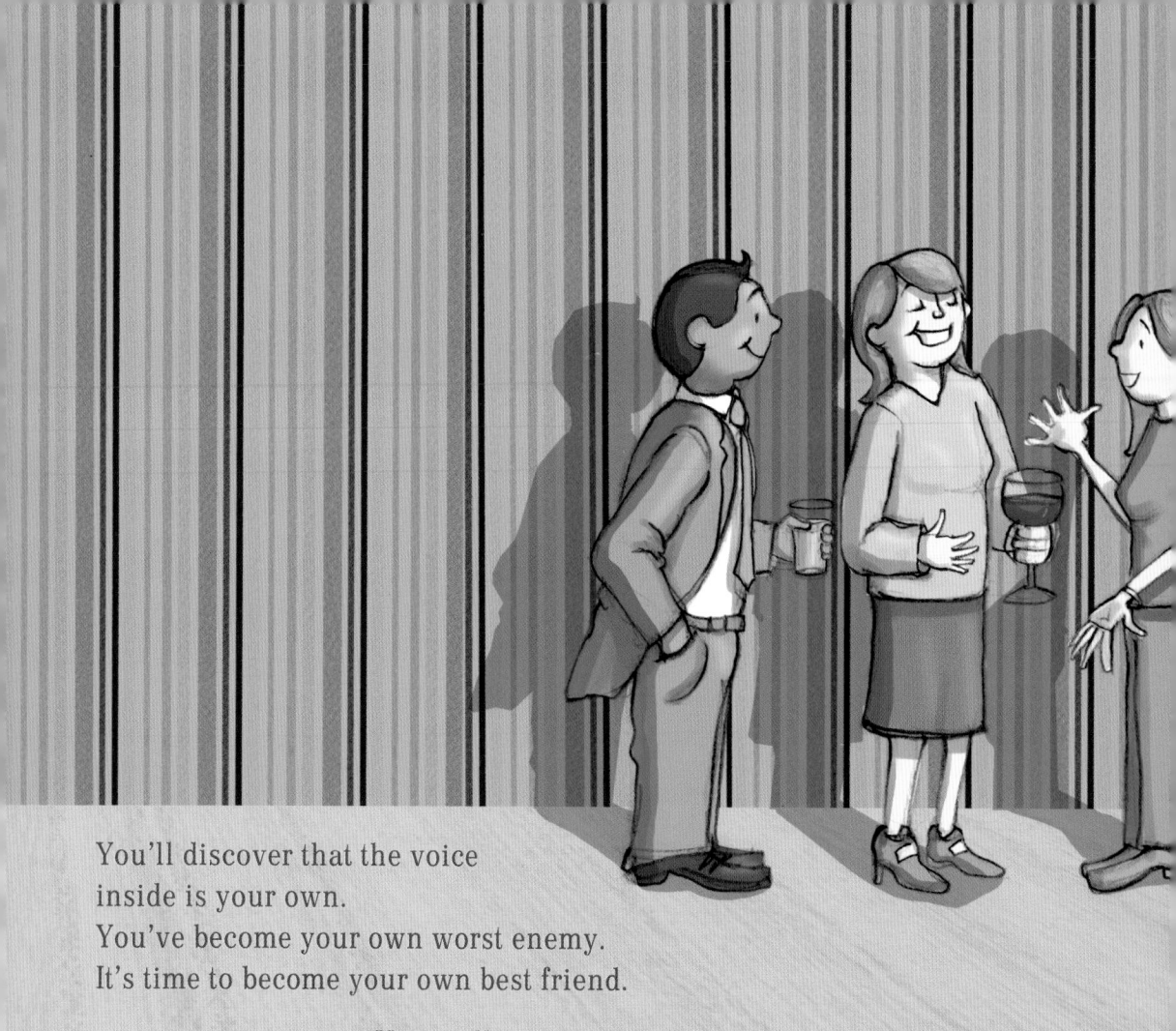

You'll discover that the voice
inside is your own.
You've become your own worst enemy.
It's time to become your own best friend.

Keep telling yourself that you are loving and loveable,
worthwhile and wonderful, interesting and inspiring.
Soon everyone else will too.

I is for INSECURITY

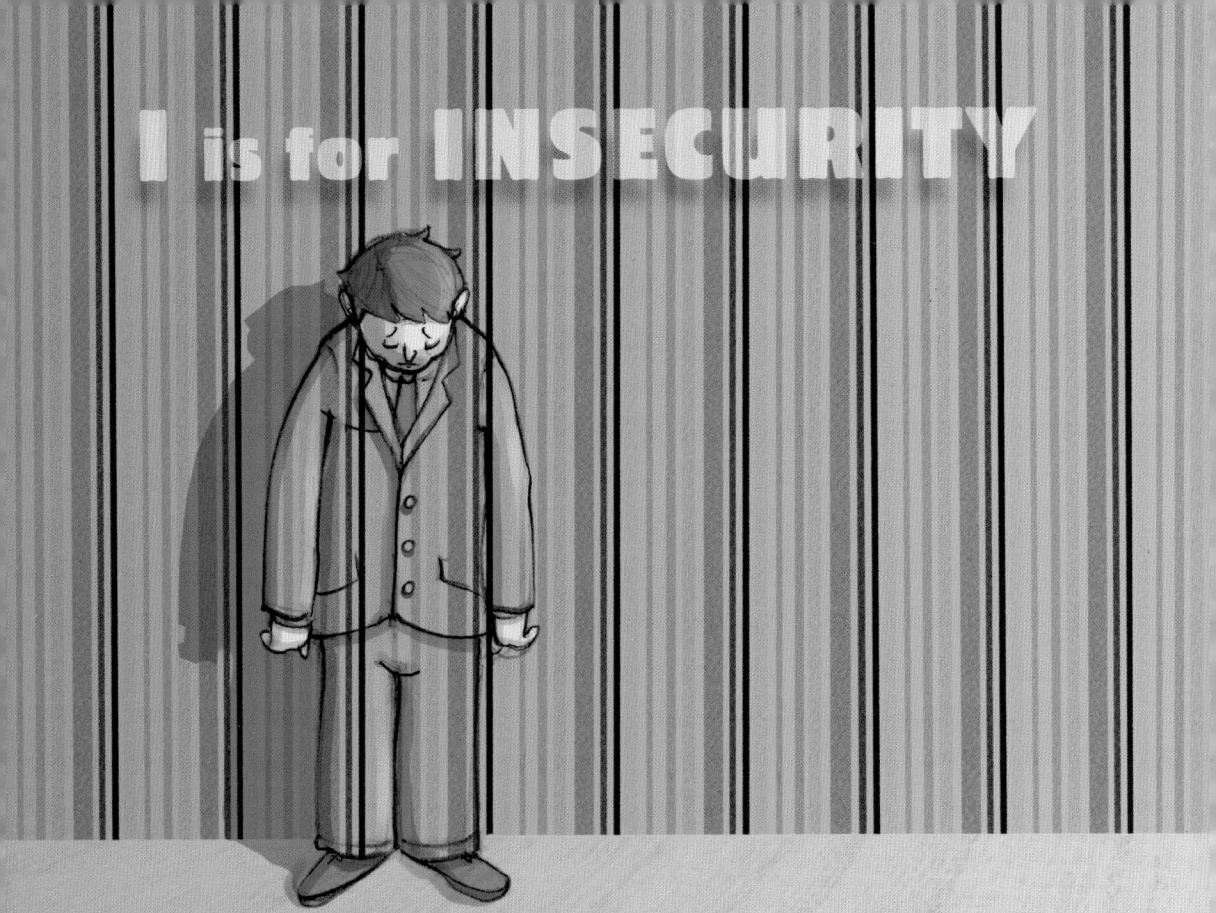

Insecurity is a dis-ease. It stems from negative self-perception.
'I'm no good'. 'I'm inadequate'. 'I'm worthless'.
It invites shyness and paranoia to the party.

Insecurity can steal our lives. But it can be overcome.
First ask yourself, who is saying these hurtful things?

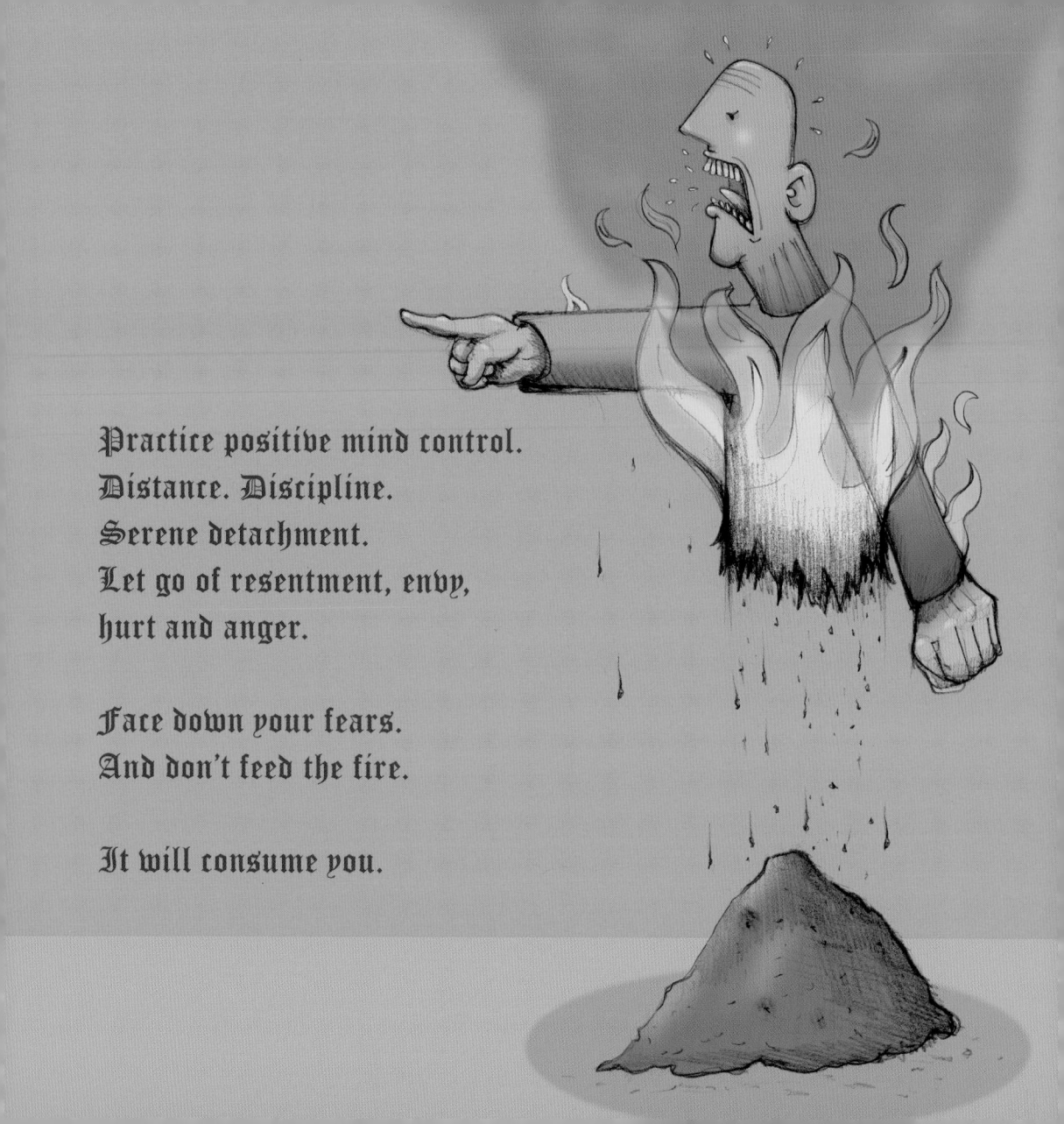

Practice positive mind control.
Distance. Discipline.
Serene detachment.
Let go of resentment, envy,
hurt and anger.

Face down your fears.
And don't feed the fire.

It will consume you.

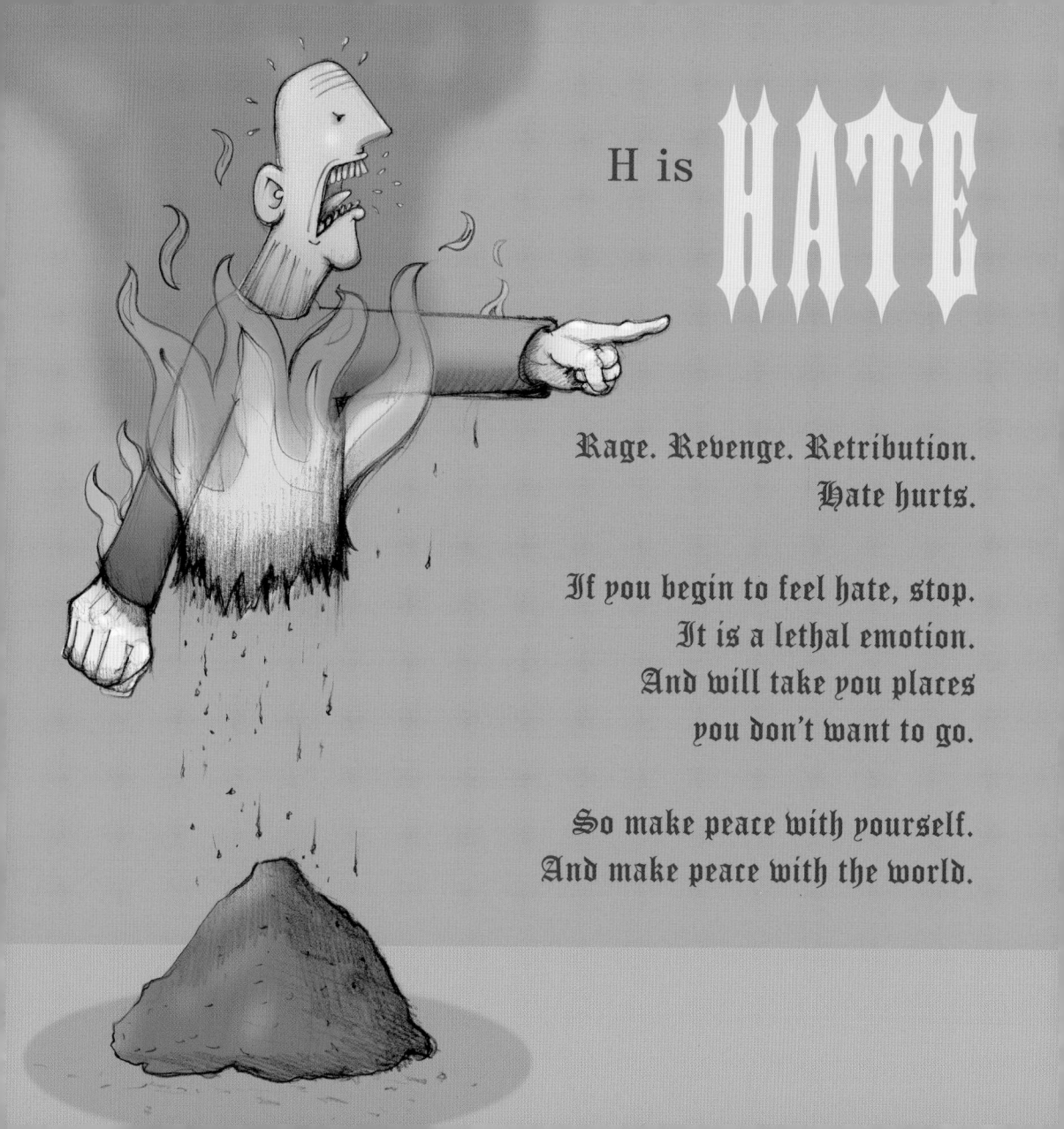

H is **HATE**

Rage. Revenge. Retribution.
Hate hurts.

If you begin to feel hate, stop.
It is a lethal emotion.
And will take you places
you don't want to go.

So make peace with yourself.
And make peace with the world.

Too much of a good thing is a bad thing.
Spiritually, the material world is immaterial.
Values, not valuables, are what define us.

Greed may make our bank balance and bellies grow,
but it shrinks our soul.

Ask yourself, how much is enough,
and how much is too much?

Sometimes the things that are supposed
to make us happy, don't.

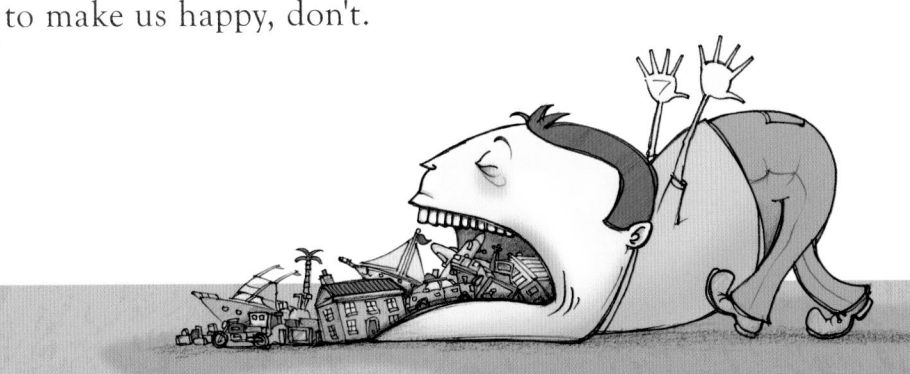

G IS
for
GREED

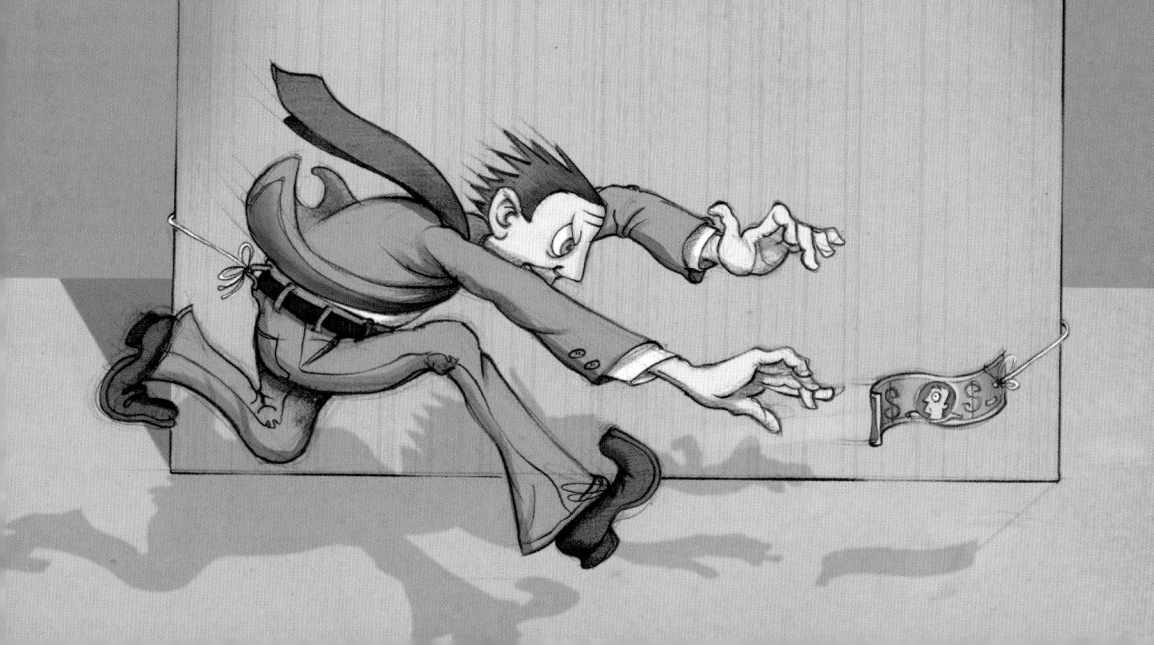

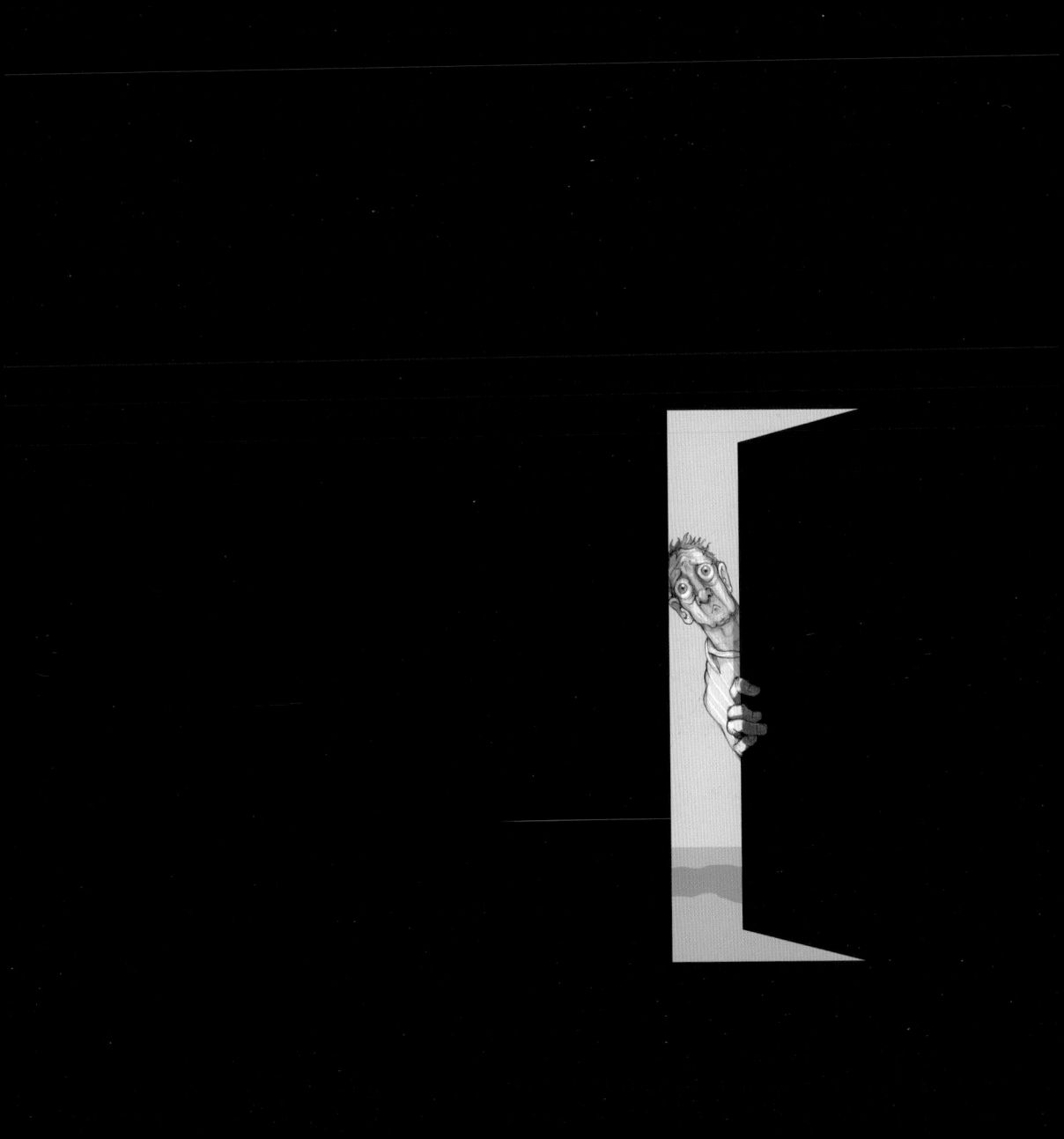

F is for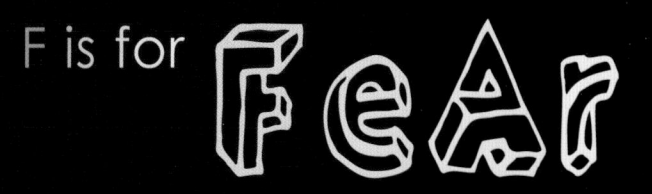

Fear holds you back.

To get over it, get into it.

Scared of heights? Jump from a plane.

Scared of spiders? Pick one up.

Scared of clowns? Paint your face.

It won't always be easy, but life will get easier.

And much less frightening.

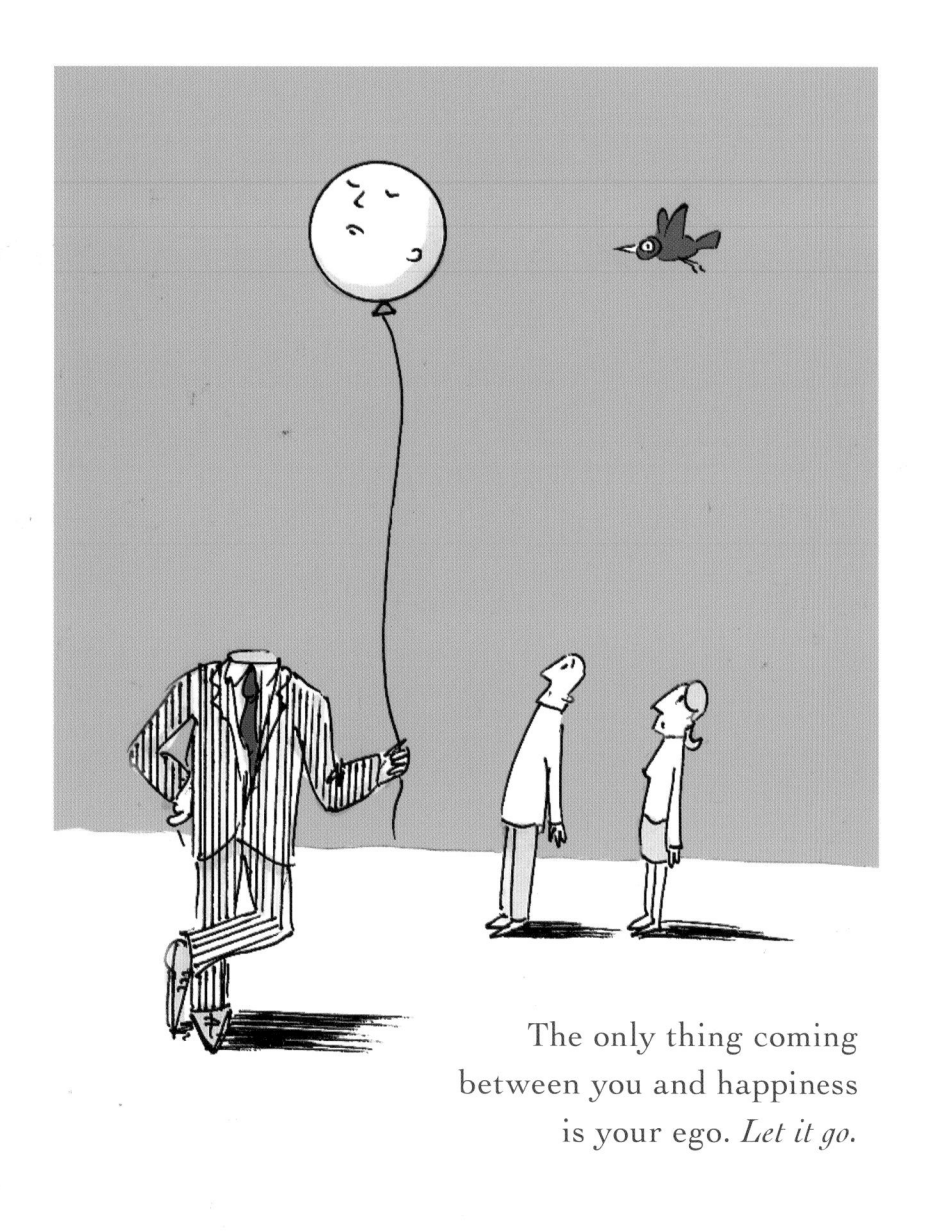

The only thing coming
between you and happiness
is your ego. *Let it go.*

E IS FOR EGO

To truly live, live for others.

To serve your best interests, serve someone else.

The less it is all about you, the more will come to you.

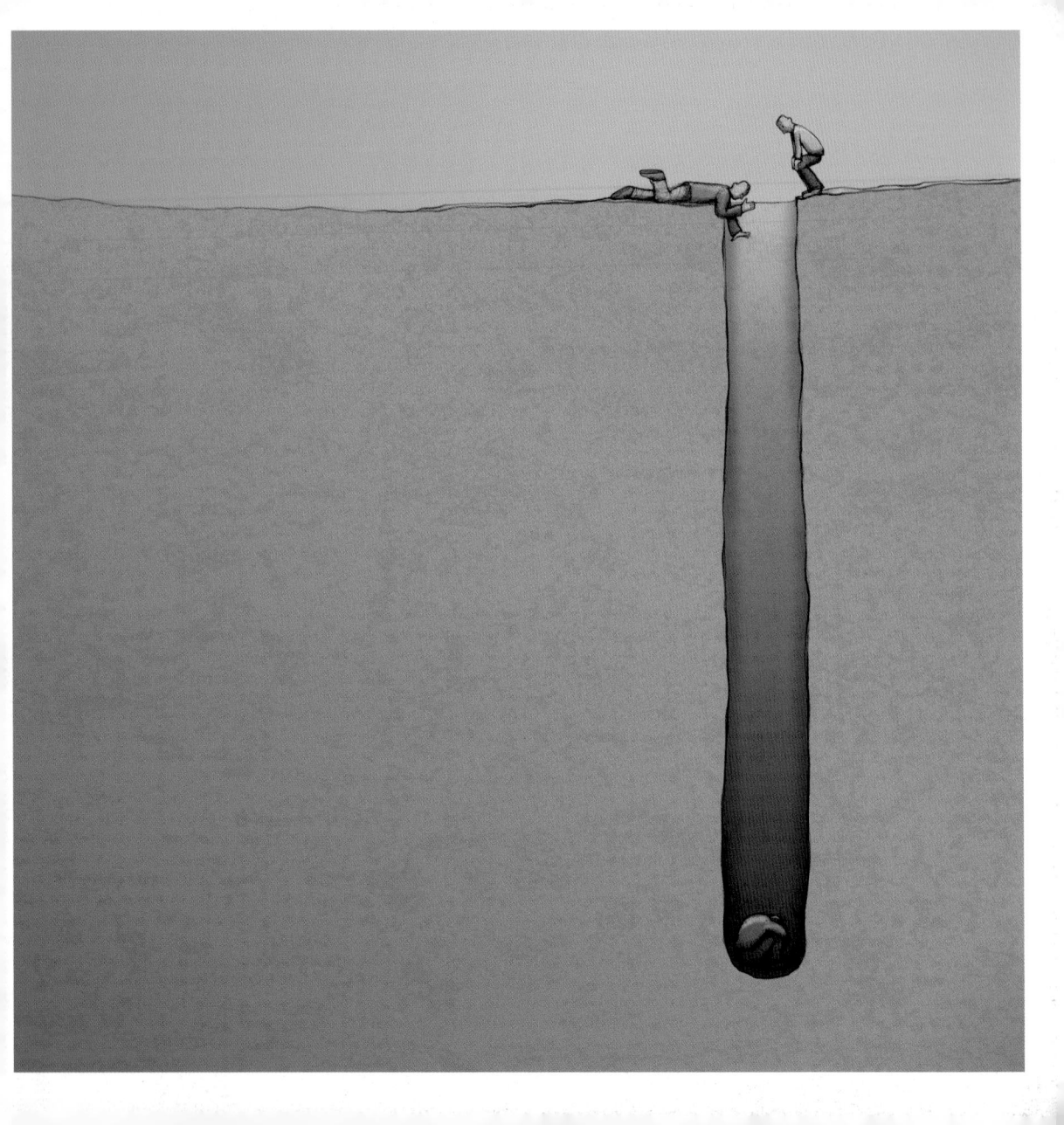

If you think you might be depressed,
the bravest thing you can do is seek help.
The only shame would be to miss out on life.

Talk to your doctor.
Find a therapist you can
trust and relate to.
Confide in your friends.

Exercise.
Eat healthily.
Rest. Meditate.
Don't self medicate.

Always remember,
this too will pass.

This too will pass

This too will pass

This too will pass

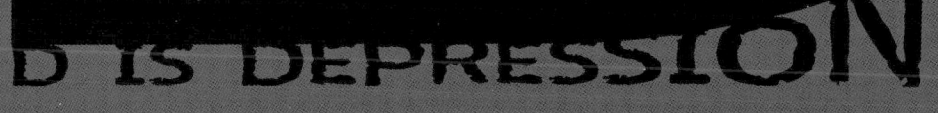

D IS DEPRESSION

Criticism tells you everything you need to know about yourself.

So listen carefully.

The faults you point out in others

are very often your own in disguise.

The way you speak about the world is the way

the world will speak about you.

How can life ever look up

if you keep putting everyone down?

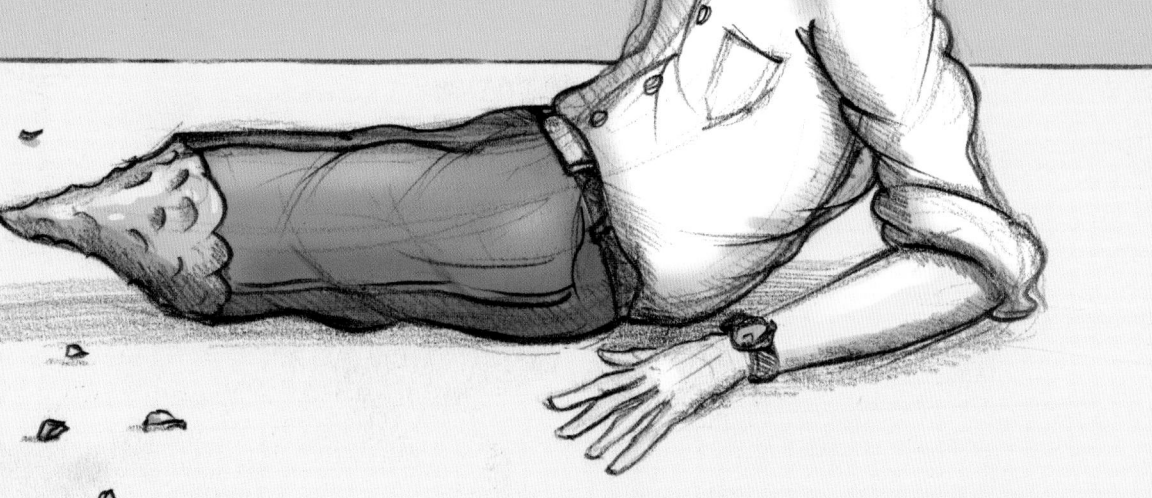

Criticism is a form of self harm. Go easy.

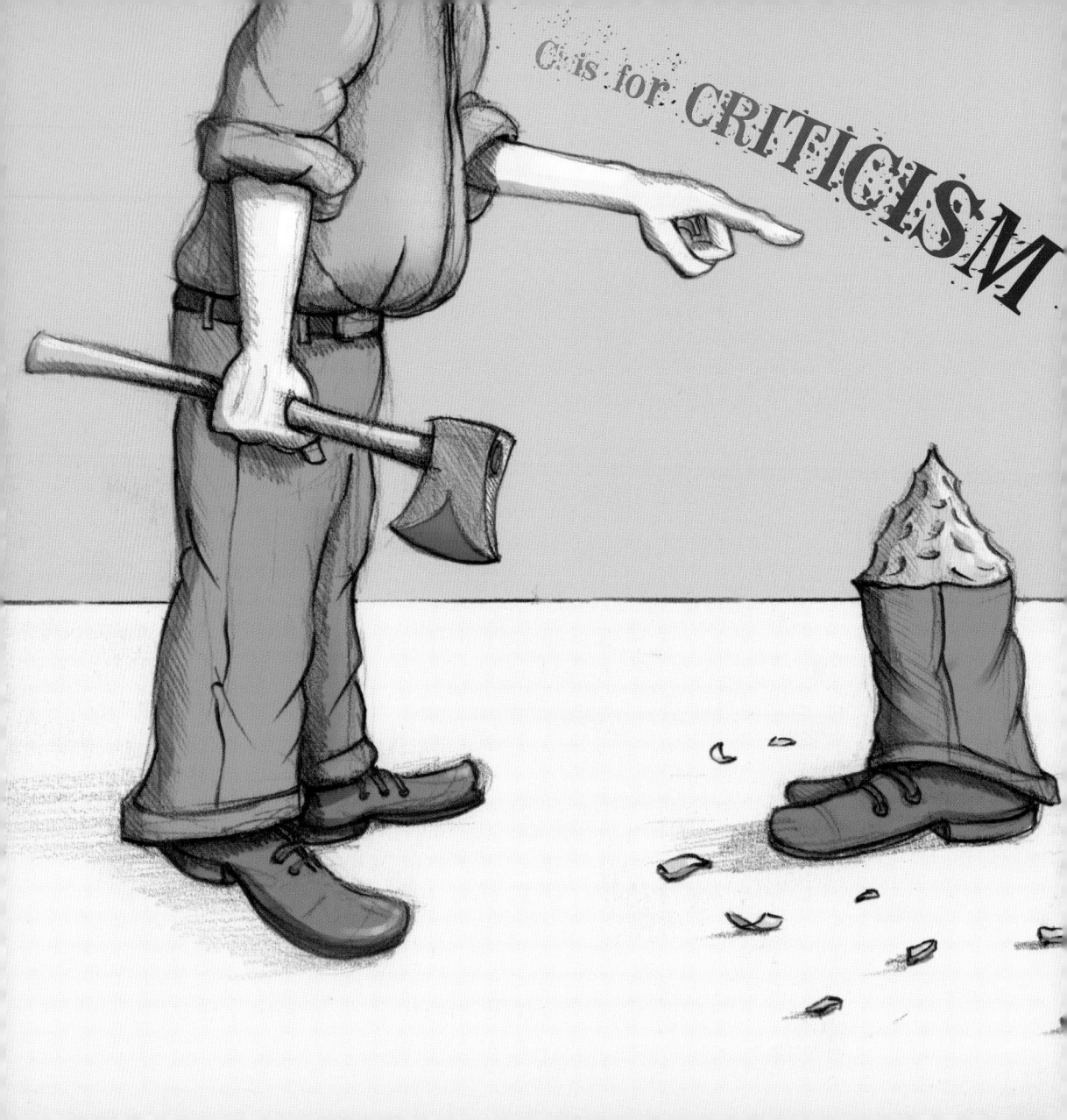

B IS FOR **BOREDOM**

BORED, RESTLESS, ANXIOUS, DISCONNECTED?

The cure is curiosity. So, try something new.

Ask a stranger to tell you a secret.

Tell your secrets to a stranger.

Experience what a kumquat tastes like.

Dress in clashing colours. Or don't dress at all.

Learn to dance. Snowboard. Paint. Sing. Juggle.

Ask a child for their advice. Take it.

Pretend that today is the last day of your life.

Or the first.

Turn off the television.

Turn on your lover.

Tune in to life.

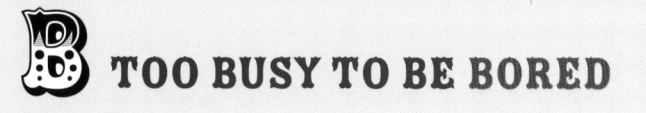 **TOO BUSY TO BE BORED**

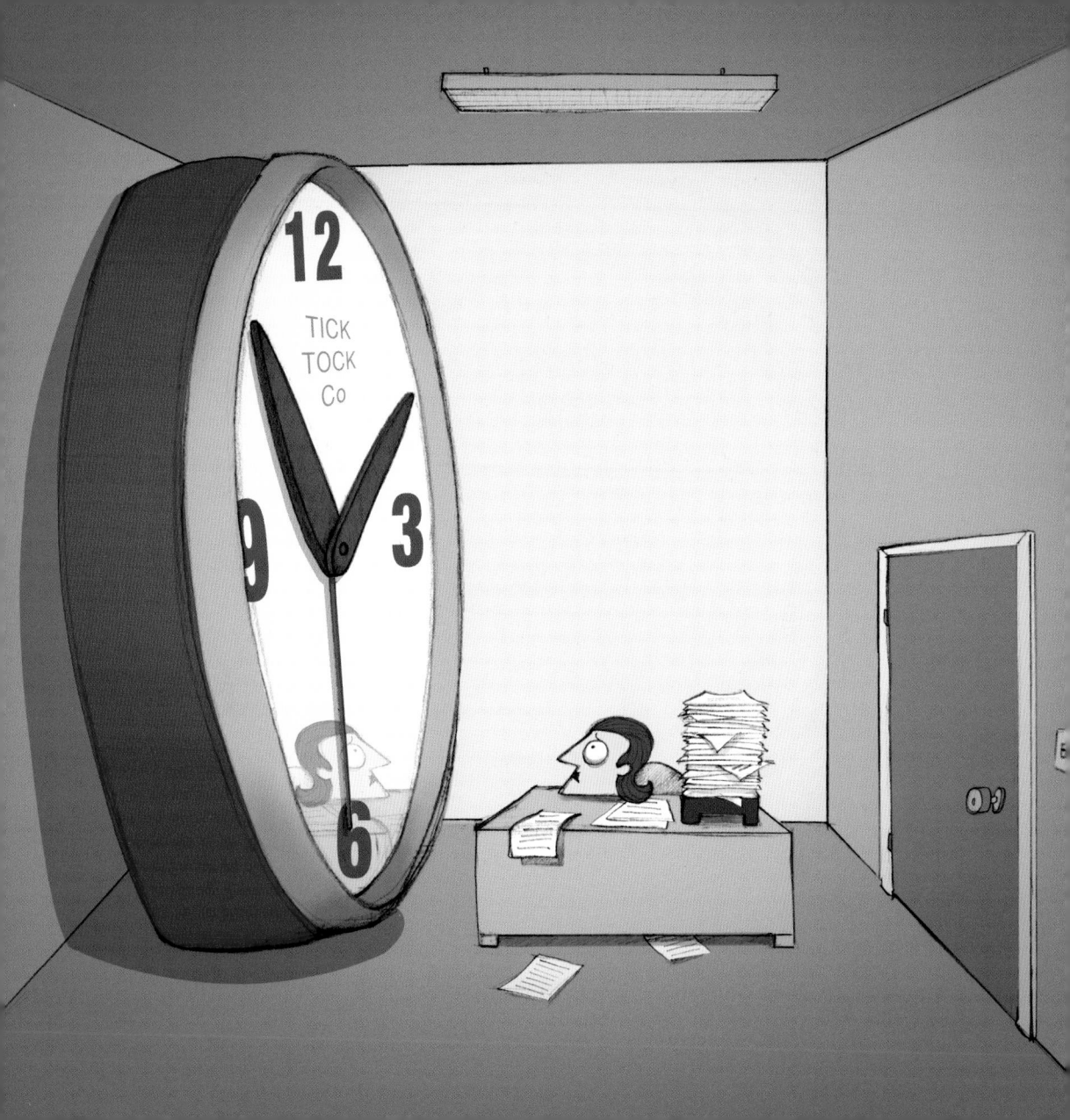

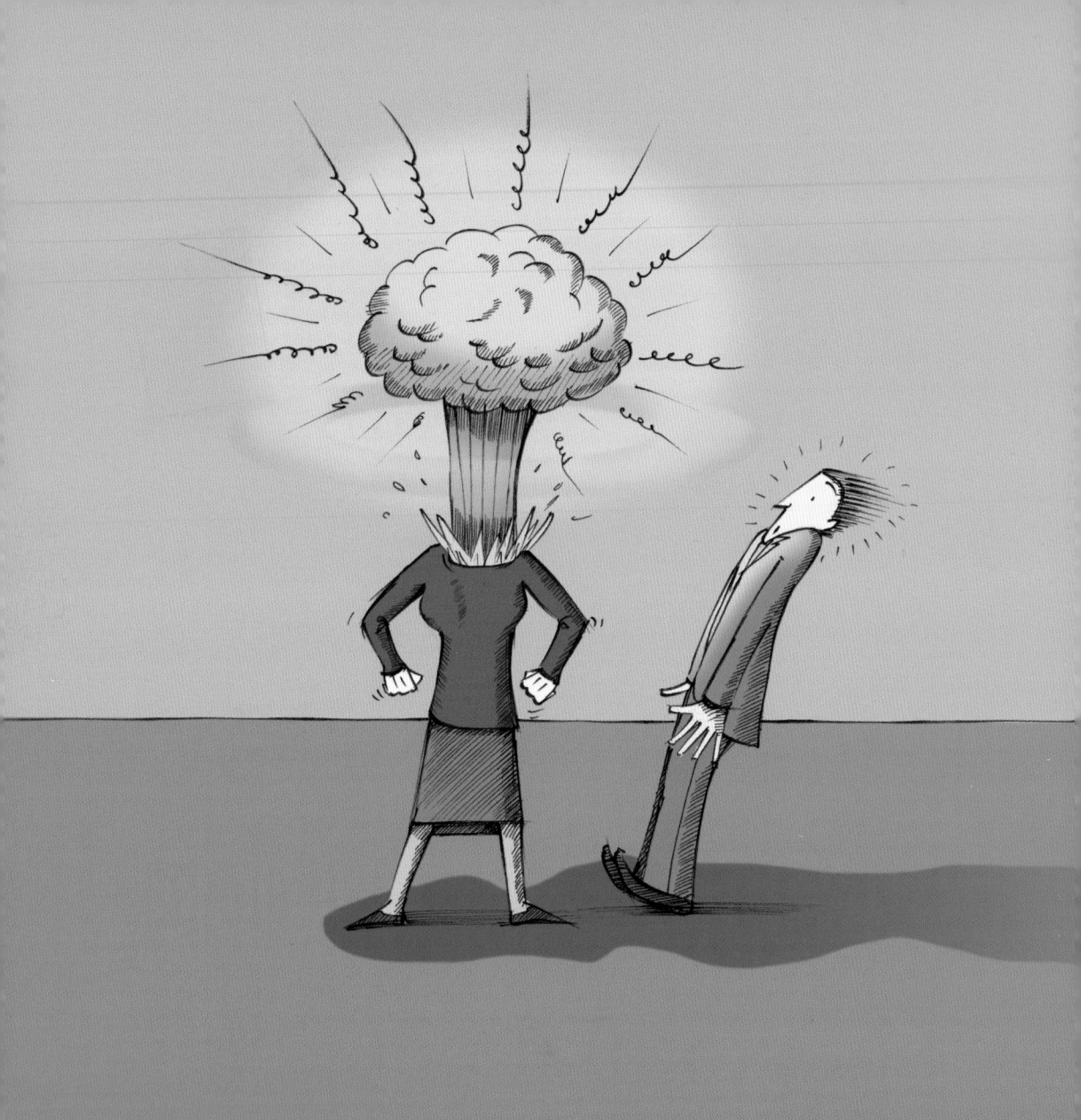

A is for

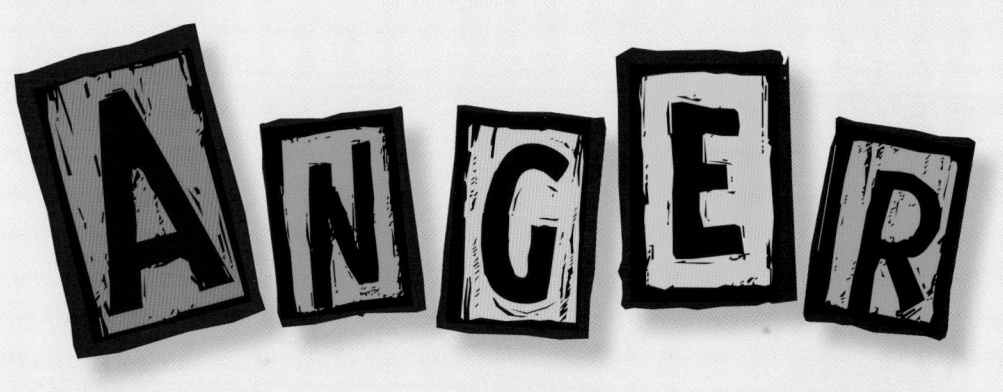

We all know what anger is.
But what makes us angry?
What fears, griefs, insecurities ... past hurts?

Understand your anger and you can overcome it.
Anger might make you enemies, but enemies
don't make you angry. Your thoughts do.

Control them and everything will be **COOL**.

By James Kerr and Matthew Johnstone

The A to Zen of Life

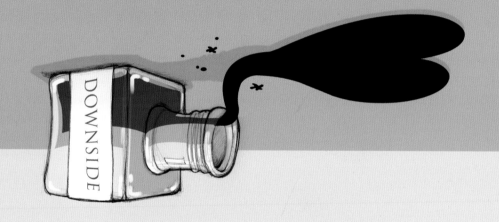

DOWNSIDE

THE ALPHABET *of the* HUMAN HEART